Fruits and Vegetables
Micronutrient and Antioxidant Quality

Vaishali Agte & Kirtan Tarwadi
*Agharkar Research Institute, Agarkar Road,
Pune - 411 004*

2012

Studium Press (India) Pvt. Ltd.

Fruits and Vegetables
Micronutrient and Antioxidant Quality

ISBN: 978-93-80012-52-0

Published by:

Studium Press (India) Pvt. Ltd.
4735/22, 2nd Floor, Prakash Deep Building
(Near Delhi Medical Association),
Ansari Road, Darya Ganj, New Delhi-110 002
Tel.: +91-11-43240200-15 (15 lines), Fax: +91-11-43240215;
jngovil@gmail.com; jngovil@hotmail.com

Printed at:

Salasar Imaging Systems, Lawrence Road, Delhi-35

Foreword

During last two decades, there has been an upsurge of knowledge regarding the micronutrients and antioxidants, particularly regarding their roles in disease and health and the use of foods rich in these phytoconstituents as nutraceutical ingredients. There have been spectacular and far reaching advances not just for the trace metals like zinc and selenium but also for vitamins E and C and for the carotenoids and flavonoids. Among different food groups, fruits and vegetables are the groups with high levels of micronutrients and antioxidants. Understanding of the functions and new roles of micronutrients and other active principles from fruits and vegetables has been considerably improved over the time. These food groups have preventive roles through multiple metabolic functions as they are integral components of antioxidant enzymes that protect organism against free radical damage. It is important to know the adequacy of micronutrient and antioxidant quality of diet to prevent oneself from possible deficiency or excess. Food science has emerged with a growing literature about fruits and vegetables imparting greater health benefits to humans. The recent focus has been on functionality of foods meaning thereby of improving quality of diet by identifying foods which boost the capacity of human body to resist disease and enhance health. These alternative medicinal approaches of increasing the intake of antioxidant and micronutrient rich foods are valuable in coping up the oxidative stress which is associated with many health disorders such as increased prevalence of diabetes, cataract, cardiovascular diseases and cancer. There is a need to develop greater awareness about consumption of protective foods such as green leafy, fruit and root vegetables, the intakes of which are far below their recommended dietary allowances. In spite of the fact that cooking losses of micronutrients are considerable, currently, the data on cooked vegetables are scanty. Majority of nutrient data books and reports available are on micronutrient contents of raw fruits and vegetables. Further, systematic data on antioxidant quality of commonly consumed fruits and vegetables both in their raw and cooked form are not available. Hence this book will cater the need of a reference book for about the individual antioxidants and micronutrients and the nutraceutical potential of fruits and vegetables available in local markets so as to emphasize their importance as inexpensive and natural food sources having health promoting properties. The book entitled *Fruits and Vegetables: Micronutrient and Antioxidant Quality* is a good attempt to bring about the latest developments on micronutrients and antioxidants as also on the health and nutraceutical aspects of fruits and vegetables. Bird's eye view for major micronutrients with detailed research based information on antioxidant micronutrients like zinc, an updated review on antioxidant and micronutrient quality of fruits and vegetables as well as effect of processing on antioxidant and micronutrient quality of fruits and vegetables has been presented. Literature review included in these chapters presents a detailed update of all essential micronutrients and antioxidants. The published data and findings covering both the positive and negative effects of antioxidants and micronutrients have been comprehensively compiled. The book contains more than 500 references taking the reader to the latest developments in the field as well as ready to use methods for assay of antioxidant and micronutrient quality. Other features of the book entitled *Fruits and Vegetables: Micronutrient and Antioxidant Quality* are that it contains laboratory generated database of fruits, uncooked and cooked vegetables commonly consumed in India, for the levels of micronutrients *viz.* thiamine, riboflavin, beta carotene, ascorbic acid, zinc, iron, copper, manganese and selenium as well as antioxidant potential indices like inhibition of lipid peroxidation, super oxide scavenging capacity, ferrous iron chelating capacity and polyphenols. Development of quality index for antioxidants and micronutrients and ranking the fruits and vegetables as poor and good sources has also been a notable feature. The book is useful as reference book to dieticians, nutritionists, food scientists, food technologists, clinicians, and as text book or additional reading material for students of home science and food technology courses. Moreover, considering the quest of knowledge by youngsters, it can attract the fitness and health conscious individuals as a ready reckoner.

I am personally delighted to see the book *Fruits and Vegetables: Micronutrient and Antioxidant Quality* coming into publication. Last and not the least of the fact is that the authors being researchers themselves have put forth extensive effort to put forth research on micronutrients and antioxidants also supported by their own published findings.

Dr. Umesh Kapil
Professor, Public Health & Nutrition
Human Nutrition Unit, All India Institute of Medical Sciences
New Delhi, India, 110029

Preface

In today's world, even a common person has become aware scientifically, towards what one should eat and what foods to avoid from the daily diet. Nutritional quality of food in earlier days was mainly judged by the contents of macronutrients *viz*. proteins, fats, carbohydrates. It was also a notion that needs for micronutrients *viz*. vitamins and essential trace metals would be automatically met when diet is sufficient in macronutrients. Then came a phase of nutritional sciences when other beneficial and harmful factors present in the food were known, which need consideration for overall health of an individual. Nevertheless, some of the truths of previous phase turned out to be myths of current time. Micronutrient inadequacies were referred as hidden hunger since body would not generate a special signal for their deficiency. Secondly, the so called antinutritional factors like polyphenols (tannins), fiber, phytates have now realized to be nutraceuticals since they have various health promoting potentials through their antioxidant activity and binding ability of harmful metabolites.

Nutritional quality of food should not only consider the contents of macro and micronutrients but also the bioavailability of nutrients, which is the extent to which the nutrient gets absorbed and utilized by the body. Further, the levels of phytonutrients having nutraceutical attributes need to be considered in judging the quality. Diversity within foods classes for the contents of nutrients and phytonutrients also need to be understood. For example, a gross advice to eat more green leafy vegetables for increasing iron intake or combating iron deficiency anemia is not appropriate. But one should know which GLVs are rich in iron and it's enhancers of bioavailability for the self or for the advocating others. Knowledge of nutrient composition of the individual foods of the diet is required for determining dietary deficiency of individuals.

There is also an emerging consensus that micronutrients and other active principles from fruits and vegetables play a preventive role in the development of chronic diseases like cancer and heart disease. Thus dietary intake of these food comodities has attained greater importance from the point of view of prevention of diseases. During the last two decades, research has brought more understanding of the roles of antioxidant vitamins such as ascorbic acid, beta carotene and trace metals like zinc, copper and selenium. Besides having multiple metabolic functions, they are integral components of antioxidant enzymes that protect human body against free radical damage. A brief summary of the important aspects of micronutrients and antioxidants has been presented and also updating the readers about latest advances about antioxidant and micronutrient quality of fruits and vegetables.

For knowing one's daily intakes of micronutrients and macronutrients, it is necessary to have a reference database of cooked foods commonly consumed in India. Currently available database on nutrients for Indian foods is by National Institute of Nutrition, Hyderabad, which is based on uncooked food analysis. Cooking and processing of foods results into loss of nutrients especially for the vitamins and antioxidants.

In an ICMR-sponsored project, a database of antioxidant activities, vitamin and mineral contents of around 100 fruits and vegetables in their uncooked and cooked states was generated for the contents of five vitamins, five minerals and for four antioxidant capacity assays. This database has been presented in this book in separate tables and this information would be certainly very useful to researchers, dieticians, doctors as also to a common man for overall health improvement. Further, an attempt has been made to develop a quality index for antioxidants and micronutrients of foods investigated by us.

List of Abbreviations

AI	:	Adequate Intake
AIDS	:	Acquired Immunodeficiency Syndrome
AMD	:	Age Related Macular Degeneration
AQI	:	Antioxidant Quality Index
ARC	:	Age Related Cataract
AREDS	:	Age Related Eye Disease Study
AVED	:	Ataxia and Vitamin E Deficiency
AVRDC	:	Asian Vegetarian Research and Development Corporation
CAT	:	Catalase
CD	:	Conjugated Diene
CHD	:	Coronary Heart Disease
CVD	:	Cardiovascular Diseases
DCPIP	:	Dichlorophenol Indophenol
DLBCL	:	Diffuse Large B-cell Lymphoma
DPPH	:	Diphenyl-1-Picrylhydrazyl
EDTA	:	Ethylene Diamine Tetra Acetic Acid
ERK	:	Extracellular Signal Regulated Kinase
EEG	:	Electroencephalogram
ESRD	:	End Stage Renal Disease
ET	:	Electron Transfer
ETs	:	Ellagitannins
FAD	:	Flavin Adenine Dinucleotide
FCR	:	Folin-Ciocalteau Reagent
FeSO4	:	Ferrous Sulphate
FICA	:	Ferrous Ion Chelating Ability
FMN	:	Flavin Mononucleotide
FNB	:	Food and Nutrition Board

FRAP	:	Ferric Reducing Antioxidant Power
GABA	:	Gamma-aminobutyric Acid
GFR	:	Glomerular Filtration Rate
GLV	:	Green Leafy Vegetables
GSH-PO	:	Glutathione Peroxidase
GSH-R	:	Glutathione Reductase
H_2O_2	:	Hydrogen Peroxide
HAT	:	Hydrogen Atom Transfer
HCl	:	Hydrochloric Acid
HDL	:	High Density Lipoproteins
HPO_3	:	Metaphosphoric Acid
ICMR	:	Indian Council of Medical Research
IDDM	:	Insulin-dependent Diabetes Mellitus
IGF	:	Intrinsic Growth Factor
ITBARS	:	Inhibition of Thiobarbituric Acid Reactive Substances
K_3FeCN_6	:	Potassium Ferricyanide
$KMNO_4$	:	Potassium Permanganate
KOH	:	Potassium Hydroxide
LDL	:	Low Density Lipoproteins
MDA	:	Malondialdehyde
MQI	:	Micronutrient Quality Index
MS	:	Multiple Sclerosis
NADH	:	Nicotinamide Adenine Dinucleotide
$NaHCO_3$	:	Sodium Bi-carbonate
NaOH	:	Sodium Hydroxide
NBT	:	Nitroblue Tetrazolium
NFκB	:	Nuclear Factor Kappa B Cells
NHL	:	Non-Hodgkin Lymphoma
NIES	:	National Institute of Environmental Sciences
NIN	:	National Institute of Nutrition
NMDAR	:	N-methyl D Aspartate Receptor
NNMB	:	National Nutrition Monitoring Bureau
NOS	:	Nitric Oxide Synthase/Species
OA	:	Osteoarthritis
ONQI	:	Overall Nutritional Quality Index
ORAC	:	Oxygen Radical Absorbance Capacity
PaA	:	Pantothenic Acid

$PbSO_4$	:	Lead Acetate
PEPCK	:	Phosphoenolpyruvate Carboxykinase
PIH	:	Pregnancy-Induced Hypertension
PLP	:	Pyridoxal Phosphate
PMS	:	Phenazine Methosulphate
PUFAs	:	Polyunsaturated Fatty Acids
Q_{10}	:	Ubiquinone
RA	:	Retinoic Acid
RDA	:	Recommended Daily Allowance
RE	:	Retinol Equivalents
RNS	:	Reactive Nitrogen Species
ROS	:	Reactive Oxygen Species
RR	:	Relative Risks
SDS	:	Sodium Dodecyl Sulphate
SELECT	:	Selenium and Vitamin E Cancer Prevention Trial
SOD	:	Superoxide Dismutase
SOSA	:	Superoxyl Scavenging Activity
TBA	:	Thiobarbituric Acid
TEAC	:	Trolox Equivalent Antioxidant Capacity
TMP	:	Thiamine Monophosphate
TPN	:	Total Parenteral Nutrition
TPP	:	Thiamin Pyrophosphate
TRAP	:	Total Radical Trapping Antioxidant Parameter
TTP	:	Thiamine Triphosphate
VTE	:	Venous Thromboembolism

Acknowledgements

The book has an indirect impact of research in the field of micronutrients and antioxidants for last 20 years, during which senior author has worked with many research students and junior colleagues. Their contribution in taking further this science of micronutrients and antioxidants is thankfully acknowledged.

Authors sincerely thank the Director, Agharkar Research Institute, Dr. Shobha Rao, HOD, Biometry and Nutrition group for their administrative support. Help from Dr. K.M. Paknikar, Head, Center for Nanobioscience and his staff for trace metal analysis by Atomic Absorption Spectrometer deserve special thanks.

Many web based search engines and web sites such as Wikipedia, Google, Entrez Pubmed, Linus Pauling Institute's Micronutrient Information Center have been referred while compiling the information on micronutrients and literature review on the subject. The access of these sites has made our work easy for which authors are thankful.

Vaishali Agte & Kirtan Tarwadi

About the Authors

Dr. Vaishali Agte

Dr. Agte has done M.Sc. in Chemistry with first class and 4th rank from Indian Institute of Technology, Powai, Mumbai in 1972. She was awarded CSIR-JRF and Ph.D in Biochemistry from Pune University in 1978 for the project '*Sparing effect of non essential amino acids on the requirements of essential amino acids in protein energy malnutrition*'. After working on projects sponsored by KVIC and BARC, she did her post doctorate research in nutritional biochemistry at Denmark during 1980. After returning back, she worked on two ICMR funded projects and then joined a faculty position as Scientist C in Agharkar Research Institute, Pune in 1982 and retired as Scientist F in 2009. As a recognized guide for Ph.D. from Pune University in Biochemistry, Biometry & Nutrition and Health sciences, she has guided 7 students for their M.Phil and Ph. D and taught nutritional biochemistry courses for M.Sc students for 4 years.

Since 1985, under various institutional and DBT, DST and ICMR funded projects, she has been doing independent research in various areas of food science and nutritional biochemistry like bioavailability of micronutrients from Indian diets and strategies to improve, micronutrient status of Indians, micronutrient interactions through cell, animal and human models, antioxidant role of zinc, studies in wild edible fruits for their antioxidant and prebiotic potential, potential of antioxidants and micronutrients from foods and herbal materials for treatment of cataract and type 2 diabetes. She has also been a recognised instructor of Art of Living and published research papers on Sudarshan Kriya. Her current areas of research are antioxidants, prebiotics, micronutrient quality of Indian foods including wheat, sorghum and green leafy vegetables, functional food development. She has 104 papers from reputed national and international journals, several chapters in the books and popular articles for magazines and newspapers to her credit.

Dr. Kirtan Tarwadi

Dr. Tarwadi is M.Sc. in Biochemistry from Maharaja Sayajirao University in 1990. She worked as ICMR – Senior Research Fellow at Agharkar Research Institute, Pune during 2000–2004. During this tenure, she accomplished her Ph.D in Biochemistry from Pune University in 2005 on a problem entitled *'Potential of antioxidants in fruits and vegetables in prevention of oxidative stress related disorders prevalent in Indians with special reference to cataract'*, under the guidance of Dr. Vaishali Agte at Agharkar Research Institute. After completing her Ph.D program, she worked as 'Principle Investigator' from December 2006 – January 2010 on the project *'Development of a nutraceutical formulation for slowing down the lens degeneration'* sponsored by DST under Women Scientist Scheme (WOS-A) under the mentorship of Dr. Vaishali Agte at Agharkar Research Institute, Pune.

Dr. Tarwadi has more than 10 years experience in area of Nutritional Biochemistry with special emphasis on food analysis involving estimation of antioxidant and micronutrient potential. She is also experienced in assessment of blood levels of oxidative stress and antioxidant activity as also micronutrient status of senile population involving diabetic and cataract patients. She is the recipient of two Young Scientist Awards, one from *'The Nutrition Society of India'* and second jointly from *'The Nutrition Society of India'* and 'The *Indian Society for Parenteral and Enteral Nutrition'*. She has attended various National and International conferences and presented many papers. She has 30 papers in national and international journals of repute to her credit. The work presented as database in this book is carried out exclusively by her under the mentorship of Dr. Vaishali Agte at Agharkar Research Institute.

Contents

1

Introduction

The doctrine 'Let food be thy medicine' espoused by Hippocrates nearly 25,000 years ago, seems to be again receiving renewed interest by the researchers. More recently, the focus has been shifted to the achievement of a balanced diet and maximization of both life expectancy and quality by identifying food ingredients that improve the capacity to resist disease and enhance health (Roberfroid, 2000). There has been a rapid increase in the oxidative stress and associated disorders such as prevalence of diabetes, cataract and cardiovascular diseases, due to rapid changes in diet and lifestyle. In adults, the prevalence of diabetes, hypertension and coronary artery disease is two to three folds greater in the urban population than in rural populations (Singh *et al.*, 1997). Nevertheless, at the individual level, natural strategies such as increased intake of antioxidant rich foods could be a valuable tool in coping up the stress.

Food science has recently emerged with a growing literature about fruits and vegetables imparting greater health benefits to humans. Fruits and vegetables which have a regular place in traditional vegetarian cuisine are being increasingly recognized for their health-advancing role. Among various types of vegetables, fruit-vegetables, roots and tubers are more popular in daily diet than the green leafy vegetables (GLV) (Plate 1).

Nutritional quality of food refers to the contents of macronutrients; proteins, fats, carbohydrates; and micronutrients; vitamins and essential trace metals, as well as bioavailability of micronutrients. There has been an emerging consensus that micronutrients and other active principles from fruits and vegetables play a preventive role in the development of chronic diseases like cancer and heart disease. Thus dietary intake of vitamins and trace minerals has attained greater importance from the point of view of prevention of diseases. The last two decades of research has brought more understanding of the functions and new roles of trace metals like zinc, copper and selenium. They have multiple metabolic functions and they are integral components of antioxidant enzymes that protect organism against free radical damage. It has also been shown that excessive exposure of essential trace elements may produce toxic effects, while deficiencies in essential trace elements can result in many pathological disturbances (Sandstead, 2000). It is therefore important to know the micronutrient contents of one's diet to prevent deficiency or excess.

Nutraceutical and functional food potential of fruits and vegetables

- There is no consensus on an exact definition of the term but functional food or medicinal food in any fresh or processed food claimed to have a health-promoting and/or disease-preventing property beyond the basic nutritional function of supplying nutrients.
- Food Science has recently emerged with a growing literature about nutraceutical aspects of fruits and vegetables imparting greater health benefits to humans.

Plate 1

Although there are some books and reports available on micronutrient contents of raw fruits and vegetables, the data on cooked vegetables are scanty. Further, systematic data on antioxidant quality of fruits and vegetables commonly consumed in India, both in their raw and cooked form are not available. Hence there is a need of a reference book to update researchers, clinicians, students and even health aware individuals about the antioxidant and micronutrient potential of fruits and vegetables available in local markets so as to emphasize their importance as inexpensive and natural sources having health-attributing properties.

OXIDATIVE STRESS AND ANTIOXIDANTS

It is ironic that oxygen, an element indispensable for life, under certain situations, has severely deleterious effects on the human body. Reactive oxygen species (ROS) is a collective term that implies to oxygen radicals and certain non-radicals, which are oxidizing agents and/or are easily converted into radicals. The oxygen radicals include superoxide ($O_2^{\cdot-}$), hydroxyl ($OH^{\cdot}$), peroxyl ($RO_2^{\cdot}$), alkoxyl ($RO^{\cdot}$) and hydroperoxyl ($HO_2^{\cdot}$), while hydrogen peroxide (H_2O_2), hypochlorus acid (HOCl), ozone (O_3) and singlet oxygen ($O_2^{\cdot}$) are among the non radicals. Generation of both reactive oxygen species results into oxidative stress (Plate 2).

Oxidative stress and antioxidants

- Reactive oxygen species also known as free radicals are the integral features of normal cellular functions
- Imbalance in oxidant-antioxidant equilibrium leads to oxidative stress
- Oxidative stress acts as an ancillary factor in pathogenesis of many non communicable diseases such as cataract, cardiovascular diseases and cancer
- Fruits and vegetables are the principal dietary sources of antioxidants to ease the load of free radicals

Plate 2

Oxidative stress is a term used to describe any situation in which ROS predominate over antioxidants; it may be due to either increased production of ROS or decreased levels of antioxidants (enzymatic and nonenzymatic) or both. Oxidative stress is a major contributing factor in certain disorders such as diabetes, cataract, cancer and cardiovascular disorder (CVD).

ESSENTIAL MICRONUTRIENTS WITH ANTIOXIDANT FUNCTIONS

Antioxidants are a group of molecules which protect living cells from the destructive consequences of powerful oxidizing intermediates that can be formed from oxygen. Situations in which pro-oxidant mechanisms within the body are more active than the antioxidant mechanisms (oxidative stress) predispose and contribute to the pathogenesis of several ailments in various organs of the body. Several nutritionally essential vitamins and trace elements have been implicated for their role in the antioxidant defense mechanism (Plate 3).

***α-tocopherol (Vitamin E)*:** Among the fat-soluble vitamins, α-tocopherol is present in all the cellular membranes and acts as a potent peroxyl radical scavenger. It acts directly with oxy radicals like $O_2^{\cdot}$, ROO·, HO· and $O_2^{\cdot-}$. It helps in glutathione recycling, and maintaining reduced glutathione levels in the lens and aqueous humor (Costagliola *et al.*, 1986).

Antioxidants and micronutrients as nutraceuticals

- *L-Ascorbic acid*: Water-soluble, cytosolic chain-breaking antioxidant; directly reacts with superoxide
- *α-Tocopherol*: Membrane bound lipid soluble chain-breaking antioxidant; reacts directly with singlet oxygen
- *β-Carotene*: Lipid soluble singlet oxygen quencher
- *Polyphenols*: Radical scavengers & metal ion chelators
- *Zinc*: Constituent of cytosolic superoxide dismutase (SOD)
- *Selenium*: Constituent of glutathione peroxidase
- *Copper*: Constituent of cytosolic SOD and ceruloplasmin
- *Iron*: Constituent of catalase
- *Manganese*: Constituent of mitochondrial SOD

Plate 3

***β-carotene*:** A pigment of plant origin, β-carotene is the most potent singlet oxygen quencher '*in vivo*'. It is the best-known and studied carotenoid due to its importance as precursor of retinol. It is found in all the cellular membranes. It exhibits strong antioxidant activity at low partial pressures of oxygen (15 torr) (Burton *et al.*, 1984). Vitamin E can protect the conjugated double bonds of β-carotene from oxidation.

***Ascorbic acid (Vitamin C)*:** Among the water-soluble vitamins, ascorbic acid is the most effective and least toxic antioxidant of mammalian systems. It has been shown to react directly with superoxide and hydroxy radicals (Machlin *et al.*, 1987). In the presence of transition metals however, it is known to provoke the formation of free radicals. The levels of ascorbate in human lenses are about thirty times higher than in the plasma, the levels of which are dependent on dietary intake of the same (Tessier *et al.*, 1998). Cataractous lenses have significantly reduced levels of ascorbate (Hankinson *et al.*, 1992), which are further compromised upon aging. On the other hand, vitamin E and β-carotene levels do not get affected in the aging lens. Next to tocopherols and carotenoids, ascorbic acid has also been a subject of interest to the researchers for intervention studies, using both animal as well as human models.

***Riboflavin*:** It is also known as vitamin $B_{2,}$ is a water-soluble B complex group of vitamin. In the body, riboflavin is primarily found as an integral component of the coenzymes, flavin adenine dinucleotide (FAD) and flavin mononucleotide (FMN) (FNB, 1998). Coenzymes derived from riboflavin are termed as flavocoenzymes, and enzymes that use a flavocoenzyme are called flavoproteins (Brody, 1999).

Glutathione reductase is a FAD-dependent enzyme that participates in the redox cycle of glutathione. The glutathione redox cycle plays a major role in protecting organisms from ROS, such as hydroperoxides.

***Thiamin*:** Thiamin occurs in the human body as free thiamin and as various phosphorylated forms: thiamin monophosphate (TMP), thiamin triphosphate (TTP), and thiamin pyrophosphate (TPP), which is also known as thiamin diphosphate. Thiamin pyrophosphate (TPP) is a required coenzyme for a small number of very important enzymes such as pyruvate dehydrogenase, β-ketoglutarate dehydrogenase, and branched chain ketoacid (BCKA) dehydrogenase and transketolase.

***Selenium*:** It is a trace element that is essential in small amounts, but like all essential elements, it is toxic at high levels. Humans and animals require selenium for the function of a number of selenium-dependent enzymes, also known as selenoproteins. At least 25 selenoproteins have been identified, but the metabolic functions have been identified for only about one-half of them (Gladyshev, 2006). Selenium-enriched garlic, broccoli, onions, and ramps (wild leeks) have been shown to reduce chemically induced tumors in rats (Whanger, 2004, 2000; Ip, 2000). Selenium-enriched vegetables are of interest because they produce some of the forms of selenium (*e.g.*, methylated forms of selenium) which may be more potent inhibitors of tumor formation than the forms currently available in supplements.

***Zinc*:** It is an essential micronutrient for all forms of life. The significance of zinc in human nutrition and public health was recognized relatively recently. Numerous aspects of cellular metabolism are zinc-dependent. Zinc plays important role in growth and development, the immune response, neurological function, and reproduction. More than 100 different enzymes depend on zinc for their ability to catalyze vital chemical reactions. Zinc-dependent enzymes can be found in all known classes of enzymes (FNB, 2001).

***Copper*:** It is an essential trace element for humans and animals. The ability of copper to easily accept and donate electrons explains its important role in oxidation-reduction (redox reactions and in scavenging free radicals (Linder and Hazegh-Azam, 1996). Copper is a critical functional component of a number of essential enzymes known as cuproenzymes such as cytochrome *c* oxidase which plays a critical role in cellular energy production, lysyl oxidase required for the cross-linking of collagen and elastin, which are essential for the formation of strong and flexible connective tissue.

***Manganese*:** It plays an important role in a number of physiological processes as a constituent of multiple enzymes and an activator of other enzymes (Nielsen, 1999). Manganese superoxide dismutase (MnSOD) is the principal antioxidant enzyme in the mitochondria. Because mitochondria consume over 90% of the oxygen used by cells, they are especially vulnerable to oxidative stress. The superoxide radical is one of the ROS produced in mitochondria during ATP synthesis. MnSOD catalyzes the conversion of superoxide radicals to hydrogen peroxide, which can be reduced to water by other antioxidant enzymes (Leach and Harris, 1987).

***Iron*:** It is a key element in the metabolism of almost all living organisms. In humans, iron is an essential component of hundreds of proteins and enzymes (Wood and Ronnenberg, 2006; Beard and Dawson, 1997). Hemoglobin and myoglobin are heme-containing proteins that are involved in the transport and storage of oxygen. Catalase and peroxidases are heme-containing enzymes that protect cells against the accumulation of hydrogen peroxide, a potentially damaging (ROS), by catalyzing a reaction that converts hydrogen peroxide to water and oxygen.

***Antioxidants*:** There are number of metabolites and phytonutrients which also have antioxidant functions. These are glutathione, carnitine, lipoic acid and polyphenols. Phenolic compounds, have received considerable attention as potentially protective factors against cancer and heart diseases because of their antioxidant potency and their ubiquity in a wide range of commonly consumed foods of plants origin. The presence of phenolic compounds in plants is important for normal growth development and defense against infection and injury. Also, phenolics may have an important effect on the oxidative stability and microbial safety in injured plants. Phenolic compounds possess one or more aromatic ring-bearing hydroxyl substituents, including their functional derivatives such as esters, methoxy compounds and glycosides. Approximately 8000 naturally occurring compounds are known which include simple phenolic, phenolic acids (benzoic and cinnamic acid derivatives), lignans, lignins, coumarins, styrylpyrones, flavonoids, isoflavonoids, stilbenes, flavonolignans and tannins. It is generally accepted that phenolic compounds behave as antioxidants as a result of the reactivity of the phenolic moiety. There are several mechanisms of antioxidant activity but it is believed that radical scavenging via hydrogen atom donation is the predominant mode. Other established antioxidant mechanisms involve radical complexing of prooxidant metals as well as quenching through electron donation and singlet oxygen quenching. Many studies have reported that phenolic compounds possess other biological activities such as antiinflammatory, antiulcer, antispasmodic, antisecretory, antiviral, antidiarrhoeal, antitumor, etc. (Gordana *et al.,* 2007).

ANTIOXIDANT DEFENSE SYSTEM OF HUMAN BODY

The intracellular defense system largely depends on antioxidant enzymes like glutathione peroxidase (GSH-PO), superoxide dismutase (SOD) and catalase (CAT) that require the antioxidant microelements. Selenium (Se) is chief constituent of GSH-PO, an enzyme important in the decomposition of hydrogen peroxide and lipid peroxides. Copper (Cu) is a constituent of cytosolic SOD, which quenches the super oxide anions, and is also an ingredient for ceruloplasmin. Zinc (Zn) is also a chief constituent of cytosolic SOD; Manganese (Mn) is a major component of mitochondrial SOD, whereas for CAT, a hemeprotein, that catalyzes the decomposition of H_2O_2, iron (Fe) is required for effective functioning. Riboflavin functions as an antioxidant as it is needed as a co-factor in the form of Flavin Adenine Dinucleotide (FAD) for glutathione reductase (GSH-R) (Duncan, 1981).

FRUITS AND VEGETABLES AS ANTIOXIDANT SOURCES

Recent studies have emerged with the health attributes for fruits and vegetables with their antioxidant action and have been implicated to offer protective role in majority of oxidative stress related disorders (Williamson *et al.,* 1997; Reddy and Bhat, 1999; Chung *et al.,* 1998; Stahl, 1998). The antioxidant properties of fruits and vegetables could be attributed to carotenoids, flavonoids, vitamins and polyphenols. Plant derived antioxidants function as oxygen quenchers, free radical scavengers, peroxide decomposers and enzyme inhibitors. The intake of antioxidant compounds present in food are now considered as important as vitamins for health promotion and protection against the damage due to oxidative stress (Fogliano, 1999; Handelman, 1999; Block, 2001).

However, due to lack of awareness, especially in slum and rural communities in India, and due to shifting to fast foods by urban elites, consumption of protective foods such as green leafy, fruit and root vegetables is far below their recommended dietary allowance (RDA)

(Praduman Kumar and Mathur, 1996). This fact is also seen in the National Nutrition Monitoring Bureau (NNMB, 1994–95) data wherein intakes of vegetables in men and women are 40% and 13% of RDA particularly in rural and tribal areas. The production and consumption of fruits and vegetables needs considerable boosting (AVRDC, 1996). Considering these facts a need was felt to understand the protective action of fruits and vegetables available in Indian markets so as to emphasize their importance in these populations as inexpensive and natural sources of micronutrients and antioxidants having health-attributing properties.

The levels of antioxidants in fruits and vegetables vary depending upon the type and agro-climatic conditions. Micronutrient contents and antioxidant capacity get affected by food processing and cooking, indicating the need for data on locally consumed cooked preparations. While the documented data on antioxidant and micronutrient potential for the cooked root and fruit-vegetables of Indian origin remain unavailable, antioxidant activity and micronutrient profile in terms of contents as well as bio-available amounts of only limited traditionally prepared GLVs is available (Agte *et al.,* 2000a, 2000b; Chiplonkar *et al.,* 1999; NIN annual report 97–98). Data on antioxidant potential for fruits and vegetables of Indian origin are still inadequate. Therefore systematic investigations were undertaken to study antioxidant potential as well as micronutrient contents covering major fruits, and GLVs, fruit vegetables root vegetables in their traditionally cooked form and uncooked form.

ASSESSMENT OF ANTIOXIDANT POTENTIAL OF FRUITS AND VEGETABLES

Several experimental systems have been reported to assess the total antioxidant capacity of individual compounds and plant extracts using *in vitro* assays. Among the reactive oxygen species (ROS), peroxide (ROO.) and super oxide (O_2^-.) are two important free radicals. The ferrous ions are also known to facilitate the free radical formation.

***Inhibition of lipid peroxidation*:** Lipid peroxidation refers to the oxidative degradation of lipids. It is the process whereby free radicals capture electrons from the lipids in cell membranes, resulting in cell damage. This process proceeds by a free radical chain reaction mechanism. It most often affects polyunsaturated fatty acids, because they contain multiple double bonds with reactive hydrogens. As with any radical reaction, the reaction consists of three major steps: initiation, propagation and termination.

Polyunsaturated fatty acids (PUFAs) are abundant in cellular membranes and in low-density lipoproteins (LDL). The PUFAs allow for fluidity of cellular membranes. A free radical prefers to steal electrons from the lipid membrane of a cell, initiating a free radical attack on the cell known as lipid peroxidation. Reactive oxygen species target the carbon-carbon double bond of polyunsaturated fatty acids. The double bond on the carbon weakens the carbon-hydrogen bond allowing for easy dissociation of the hydrogen by a free radical. A free radical will steal the single electron from the hydrogen associated with the carbon at the double bond. In turn this leaves the carbon with an unpaired electron and hence becomes a free radical. In an effort to stabilize the carbon-centered free radical molecular rearrangement occurs. The newly arranged molecule is called a conjugated diene (CD). The CD then very easily reacts with oxygen to form a peroxy radical. The peroxy radical captures an electron from another lipid molecule in a process called propagation. Nevertheless, many natural products like fruits and vegetables have ability to inhibit lipid peroxidation resulting into partially or completely save the cells from possible damage.

***Superoxyl scavenging activity*:** Superoxide anions are formed when oxygen (O_2) acquires an additional electron, leaving the molecule with only one unpaired electron. Within the mitochondria $O_2^{-}\cdot$ is continuously being formed. Superoxide anion radical ($O_2^{\cdot -}$) is one of the strongest reactive oxygen species among the free radicals that are generated first after oxygen is taken into living cells. $O_2^{-}\cdot$ changes to other harmful reactive oxygen species and free radicals such as hydrogen peroxide and hydroxyl radical. Superoxyl scavenging activity of foods is therefore important biomarker of antioxidant potential.

***Ferrous ion chelating ability*:** Iron is a potent generator of oxidative damage whose levels increase with age, potentially exacerbating age-related diseases. It can cause oxidative stress since ferrous iron (Fe^{+2}) reacts with H_2O_2 in the Fenton reaction to produce the highly reactive hydroxyl radical, which can damage proteins, lipids, and nucleic acids. In this context, the ability of fruits and vegetables to chelate the ferrous iron carries significance.

IMPORTANCE OF DATA ON MICRONUTRIENT AND ANTI-OXIDANT QUALITY

Vegetables contain not only the nutritional antioxidants but also a great quantity of non-nutritional antioxidants, such as flavonoids, flavone, and polyphenol compounds. Many studies have indicated that a frequent intake of cruciferous vegetables, such as broccoli, cauliflower, leaf mustard, cabbage, Chinese broccoli, and turnip, could protect against cancer. (Plate 4-6)

Among various fruits and vegetables available in the Indian markets, 15 root vegetables, 12 fruit vegetables, 30 fruits and 30 GLV were identified as the commonly consumed types. Their frequent availability and demand in the market were taken to be the indicators of their popularity.

Active principles in fruits and vegetables

- *Carotenoids*: α/β/γ carotene, lycopene, lutein, zeaxanthin, cryptoxanthin
- *Flavonoids & Polyphenols*: quercetin, caffeic acid, ferulic acid, gallic acid, chlorogenic acid, tannic acid and ellagic acid
- *Organic acids*: malic, citric, hydroxy citric
- *Glycans*: free sugars, oligosaccharides, cellulose, hemicellulose
- *Enzyme inhibitors against*: α amylase, β glucosidase, tyrosinase, proteases
- *Vitamins*: thiamine, riboflavin, niacin, pyridoxin, folic acid, ascorbic acid
- *Minerals*: *Ca, Mg, Na, Mg, K, P*
- *Trace minerals*: *Fe, Zn, Cu, Mn, Se, I*

Plate 4

All the fruits and vegetables, screened for the present study, were procured from market fresh, cleaned and edible portions were collected.

Fruits and vegetables

Health-attributes

- Rich source of bioactive principles with implications as 'nutraceutical package'
- Conferred the status of functional foods for their health promoting role

Intake among Indians

- Low intake of fruits in Indians due to lack of awareness and affordability
- Intake of vegetables among rurals as low as 13% & among urbans as low as 25% of the recommended daily allowance (RDA)

Plate 5

Initially all the foods were analyzed for their antioxidant potential in the raw states. Later the vegetables alone (without any additions) were pressure cooked for 5 minutes at 15 lb. pressure and homogenized in a blender to estimate the antioxidant activity in their cooked form. This way of cooking was chosen because it does not involve addition of oil and other food ingredients, which may also have antioxidant activities.

For knowing one's daily intakes of micronutrients and antioxidants, it is necessary to have a reference database of cooked foods commonly consumed in India. Currently available database on nutrients for Indian foods is by National Institute of Nutrition, Hyderabad, which is based on raw food analysis (NIN 2000). It is difficult to use these values for cooked foods' consumption due to use of multiple food ingredients and presence of water in the cooked foods. Secondly, cooking and processing of foods results into loss of many vitamins. It is necessary to have values of vitamin contents in cooked or read-to-eat foods. Such datasets are scarce especially for Indian foods, which has a large variety of items, cooking processes and food combinations. This further stresses the need for a comprehensive database on micronutrient contents of cooked foods to assess the dietary micronutrient status of an individual.

Major nutraceutical effects of fruits and vegetables

- Antioxidant (reducing oxidative stress)
- Anticarcinogen (cancer preventive)
- Hepato-protective (liver protective)
- Antidiabetic (control of diabetes)
- Cardio-protective (heart protective)
- Prebiotic (increase in growth of good bacteria)
- Antibacterial (reduction in harmful bacteria)

Plate 6

In the ICMR-sponsored project, database of vitamin and mineral contents as well as antioxidant potential of around 90 cooked vegetables and 120 raw fruits and vegetables were generated. This database have been presented in this book in separate tables and this information would be certainly useful to researchers, dieticians, doctors and also common man. This will be useful as tips for health improvement and to judge the levels of these factors in one's daily diet.

***Audience/readership*:** The book would be useful to nutritionists, food scientists, home science students, graduate and post graduate of medical colleges, medical and health professionals, policy makers of child and women health as also the homemakers.

REFERENCES

Agte V, Indumadhavi M, Kakade V, Tarwadi K, and Chiplonkar S 2000. Role of diet related habits and cooking practices on bioavailability of iron, copper and zinc and status of iron in vegetarians. Proceedings of TEMA-10, pp. 65–67.

Agte V, Tarwadi K, Mengale S, and Chiplonkar S 2000. Potential of traditionally cooked green leafy vegetables as natural sources for supplementation of 8 micronutrients in vegetarian diets. *J. Food Compo. Anal.* 13: 885–891.

AVRDC Report 1996. Combating micronutrient deficiency through vegetables Centerpoint pp. 4–5.

Beard J, and Dawson H Iron 1997. *In*: O'Dell BL, and Sunde RA, *Eds*. Handbook of nutritionally essential minerals. New York: Marcel Dekker, Inc, pp. 275–334.

Block G, 2001. Which plasma antioxidants are more related to fruit and vegetable consumption? *American Journal of Epidemiology* 12: 1113–1118.

Brody T, 1999. Nutritional Biochemistry. 2nd *Ed*. San Diego: Academic Press.

Burton W, and Ingold KU 1984. Beta carotene: An unusual type of lipid antioxidant. *Science* 224: 569–573.

Chiplonkar S, Tarwadi K, Kavedia R, Mengale S, Paknikar K, and Agte V 1999. Fortification of vegetarian diets for increasing bioavailable iron density using green leafy vegetables. *Foods Inter.* 32: 169–174.

Chung K, Weichang I, and Johnson M 1998. Are tannins a double edged sword in biology and health? *Trends in Food Science and Technology* 4: 168–175.

Costagliola C, Luliano G, Menzione M, Rinaldi E, Vito P, and Aurricchio G 1986. Effect of vitamin E on glutathione content in red cells, aqueous humor and lens of humans and other species. *Exp. Eye Res.* 43: 905–914.

Duncan G, 1981. Mechanisms of cataract formation in the human lens. London: Academic Press, Inc., U.K.

Fogliano V, Verde V, Randazzo G, and Ritieni A 1999. Method for measuring antioxidant activity and its application to monitoring the antioxidant capacity of wines. *J. Agri. Food Chem.* 47: 1035–1040.

Food and Nutrition Board, 1998. Institute of Medicine. Riboflavin. Dietary Reference Intakes: Thiamin, Riboflavin, Niacin, Vitamin B_6, Vitamin B_{12}, Pantothenic Acid, Biotin, and Choline. Washington D.C.: National Academy Press pp. 87–122.

Food and Nutrition Board, 2001. Institute of Medicine. Zinc. Dietary reference intakes for vitamin A, vitamin K, boron, chromium, copper, iodine, iron, manganese, molybdenum, nickel, silicon, vanadium, and zinc. Washington, DC: National Academy Press; 442–501.

Gladyshev V, 2006. Selenoproteins and selenoproteomes. *In*: Hatfield DL, Berry MJ, and Gladyshev VN, *Eds*. Selenium: Its molecular biology and role in human health. 2nd ed. New York: Springer, pp. 99–114.

Gordana S, Æetkoviæ J, Èanadanoviæ-B, *et al.* 2007. Cvetkoviæ Antioxidant potential, lipid peroxidation inhibition and antimicrobial activities of *Satureja montana* L. subsp. *kitaibelii*. extracts *Int. J. Mol. Sci.* 8: 1013–1027.

Handelman G, Cao G, Walter M, *et al.* 1999. Antioxidant capacity of oat extracts. Inhibition of low-density lipoprotein oxidation and oxygen radical absorbance capacity. *J. Agri. Food Chem.* 47: 4886–4893.

Hankinson SE, Stampfer MJ, and Seddon JM 1992. Nutrient intake and cataract extraction in women: A prospective study. *Br. Med. J.* 305: 335–339.

Ip C, Birringer M, Block E, *et al.* 2000. Chemical speciation influences comparative activity of selenium-enriched garlic and yeast in mammary cancer prevention. *J. Agric. Food Chem.* 48(6): 2062–2070.

Leach R, and Harris E 1997. Manganese. *In*: O'Dell BL, and Sunde RA, *Eds.* Handbook of nutritionally essential minerals. New York: Marcel Dekker, Inc; 335–355.

Linder M, and Hazegh-Azam M 1996. Copper biochemistry and molecular biology. *Am. J. Clin. Nutr.* 63(5): 797S–811S.

Machlin L, and Bendich A 1987. Free radical tissue damage: Protective role of antioxidant micronutrients. *FASEB J.* 1: 441–445.

National Institute of Nutrition, 1997–98. Annual Report, NIN, ICMR, Hyderabad.

National Nutrition Monitoring Bureau (NNMB) 1994–95. National Institute of Nutrition NIN, ICMR, Hyderabad.

Nielsen FH, 1999. Ultratrace minerals. *In*: Shils M, Olson JA, Shike M, and Ross AC, *Eds*. Modern Nutrition in Health and Disease. 9th ed. Baltimore: Williams & Wilkins pp. 283–303.

Nutritive Value of Indian Foods 2000. *Edited* by C Gopalan, BV Ramashastri and SC Balasubramanian. National Institute of Nutrition NIN, ICMR, Hyderabad.

Praduman Kumar, and Mathur VC 1996. Structural changes in the demand for food in India. *Ind. J. Agric. Economics* 51: 664–673.

Reddy G, and Bhat K 1999. Protection against UVB inactivation (*in vitro*) of rat lens enzymes by natural antioxidants. *Molecular and Cellular Biochem.* 194: 41–45.

Roberfroid MB 2000. Prebiotics and probiotics: are they functional foods? *Am. J. Clin. Nutr.* 71(6 Suppl): 1682S–7S; discussion 1688S–90S.

Sandstead H, and Leslie M Klevay 2000. History of Nutrition Symposium: Trace Element Nutrition and Human Health[1]. *Journal of Nutrition* 130: 483S–484S.

Singh RB, Niaz MA, and Ghosh S 1997. Effect on central obesity and associated disturbances of low-energy, fruit- and vegetable-enriched prudent diet in north Indians. *Postgrad Med. J.* 70: 895–900.

Stahl W, 1998. Carotenoid mixtures protect multilamellar liposomes against oxidative damage: synergistic effects of lycopene and lutin. *FEBS Letters* 427: 305–308.

Tessier F, Moreaux V, and Birlouez-Aragon B 1998. Decrease in vitamin C concentration in human lenses during cataract progression. *Internat. J. Vit. Nutr. Res.* 68: 309–315.

Whanger PD, 2004. Selenium and its relationship to cancer: an update. *Br. J. Nutr.* 91(1): 11–28.

Whanger PD, Ip C, Polan CE, Uden PC, and Welbaum G 2000. Tumorigenesis, metabolism, speciation, bioavailability, and tissue deposition of selenium in selenium-enriched ramps (*Allium tricoccum*). *J. Agric. Food Chem.* 48(11): 5723–5730.

Williamson Gary, M Susan DuPont, Su Wanigatunga, Robert K Heaney, Stephen RR Musk, G Roger Fenwick, and Michael JC Rhodes 1997. Induction of glutathione S-transferase activity in hepG2 cells by extracts of fruits and vegetables. *Food Chem.*, 2: 157–160.

Wood RJ, and Ronnenberg AG 2006. Iron. *In*: Shils ME, Shike M, Ross AC, Caballero B, and Cousins RJ, *Eds*. Modern Nutrition in Health and Disease. 10th ed. Philadelphia: Lippincott Williams & Wilkins pp. 248–270.

2

Importance of Vitamins in Our Diet

Vitamins are organic molecules functioning to facilitate an essential biochemical reaction necessary for growth, vitality and the normal functioning of our body. The term vitamin, is conditional both on the circumstances and specific for the organisms. For example, ascorbic acid is a vitamin for humans, but not for most other animals. Vitamins are essentially classified by their biological and chemical activity, not by their structure. Thus, each "vitamin" refers to a number of vitamer compounds that all exhibit the biological activity associated with a particular vitamin to a variable extent. Such a set of chemicals are grouped under an alphabetized vitamin "generic descriptor" title, such as "vitamin A", which includes the compounds retinal, retinol, and four known carotenoids. Vitamers by definition are convertible to the active form of the vitamin in the body, and are sometimes inter-convertible to one another, as well. Thirteen vitamins are presently universally recognized (Plate 7).

***Fat-soluble vitamins*:** These are vitamins A, D, E, and K. These vitamins are absorbed, transported, metabolized and stored along with fat. The fat soluble vitamins function as regulators for specific metabolic activity.

***Water-soluble vitamins*:** The water-soluble vitamins are ascorbic acid (vitamin C), and those of the B-complex group: thiamin (B_1), riboflavin (B_2), nicotinic acid (B_3), pantothenic acid (B_5) pyridoxine (B_6), biotin (B_7), folic acid (B_9) and cyanocobalamin (B_{12}) which function mainly as coenzymes and some as antioxidants.

Vitamin content of fruits and vegetables (Tarwadi and Agte, 2007)				
Food class	*Ascorbic acid mg/100 g*	*β-carotene μg/100 g*	*Riboflavin mg/100 g*	*Thiamine mg/100 g*
Fruit veg. cooked	5.5 ± 3.92	17 ± 20.6	0.02 ± 0.01	0.02 ± 0.01
Root veg. cooked	4.0 ± 3.38	56 ± 164	0.15 ± 0.01	0.01 ± 0.01
GLV cooked	10.9 ± 14.58	1138 ± 65.1	0.08 ± 0.02	0.03 ± 0.01
Fruits (fresh)	38 ± 318	66 ± 1133	0.14 ± 0.12	0.15 ± 0.11
Fruit veg. uncooked	18.6 ± 25.59	50 ± 45.3	0.02 ± 0.01	0.03 ± 0.01
Root veg. uncooked	9.4 ± 7.29	126 ± 308.7	0.02 ± 0.01	0.02 ± 0.01
GLV uncooked	30.1 ± 33.4	3324 ± 1886.6	0.10 ± 0.02	0.03 ± 0.01

Plate 7

VITAMINS WITH ANTIOXIDANT FUNCTIONS

Vitamin A or Retinol

Vitamin A is a generic term for a large number of related compounds. Vitamin A is a fat-soluble vitamin that occurs in two forms in nature. Retinol (an alcohol) and retinal (an aldehyde) are often referred to as preformed vitamin A. Retinal can be converted by the body to retinoic acid. Retinol, retinal, retinoic acid, and related compounds are known as retinoids. Vitamin A can be found in vegetables in the form of beta-carotene or provitamin A. This form is found in plants and is the precursor of the actual vitamin. Beta-carotene has to be converted in the body in order to be used by it. Fat and bile are needed for the conversion. The liver regulates the blood level of vitamin A. It needs a special protein carrier to be transported throughout the body. An adequate protein and fat intake is required for a good absorption of vitamin A.

***Units of measurement and RDA*:** Vitamin and mineral amounts are usually expressed in milligrams (mg) or micrograms (mcg). Vitamin A values are expressed in different ways. The nutrient was originally measured in I.U (international unit) but in 1974 the United States began using a measurement called Retinol Equivalents (REs). One IU is equivalent to 0.3 microgram (mcg) of retinol, and one mcg of retinol is equivalent to 3.33 IU of retinol. 1 RE = 1 mcg. of retinol, 1 RE = 6 mcg. of beta-carotene. The RDA for vitamin A is 2,300 IU/day for women and 3,000 IU/day to support normal gene expression, immune function, and vision.

Functions of vitamin A

***Vision*:** Retinol is transported to the retina via the circulation and accumulates in retinal pigment epithelial cells in the form of retinyl esters, which can be stored. When needed, retinyl esters are hydrolyzed and isomerized to form 11-cis-retinol, which can be oxidized to form 11-cis-retinal. It can be shuttled across the inter photoreceptor matrix to the rod cell where it binds to a protein called opsin to form the visual pigment, rhodopsin (also known as visual purple). Rod cells with rhodopsin can detect very small amounts of light, making them important for night vision. This isomerization triggers a cascade of events, leading to the generation of an electrical signal to the optic nerve. The nerve impulse generated by the optic nerve is conveyed to the brain where it can be interpreted as vision (Gropper, 2009). Inadequate retinol available to the retina results in impaired dark adaptation which is also popularly known as 'night blindness' (Semba, 1999; Sommer, 2008).

***Immunity*:** Vitamin A is commonly known as the anti-infective vitamin, because it is required for normal functioning of the immune system (Scultink, 2002). Retinol and its metabolites are required to maintain its integrity and function (Thompson *et al.*, 2005). Vitamin A and retinoic acid (RA) play a central role in the development and differentiation of white blood cells, such as lymphocytes, which play critical roles in the immune response.

***Growth and development*:** Retinol and retinoic acid (RA) are essential for embryonic development (Scultink, 2002). During fetal development, RA functions in limb development and formation of the heart, eyes, and ears (Mohsen *et al.*, 2008). Additionally, RA has been found to regulate expression of the gene for growth hormone.

***Red blood cell production*:** Stem cells are dependent on retinoids for normal differentiation into red blood cells. Additionally, vitamin A appears to facilitate the mobilization of iron from storage sites to the developing red blood cell for incorporation into hemoglobin, the oxygen carrier in red blood cells (Gropper, 2009; Stone bred, 1995).

Sources of vitamin A

Cod liver oil is the richest source of vitamin A. Animal products are also good sources of vitamin A. Vegetarians need to increase the intake of beta-carotene (the precursor of vitamin A) to ensure their intake in vitamin A. Beta-carotene is found in abundance in bright yellow, orange, red and dark green fruits and vegetables. Carrots, mango (ripe variety), spinach, broccoli, kale, collard are also some of the rich sources of the vitamin.

Deficiency

Vitamin A deficiency is common in developing countries but rarely seen in developed countries. Approximately 250,000 to 500,000 malnourished children in the developing world go blind each year from a deficiency of vitamin A (Semba, 1999; Sommer, 2008). Night blindness is one of the first signs of vitamin A deficiency (Scultink, 2002; Stone bred, 1995). Vitamin A deficiency contributes to blindness by making the cornea very dry and damaging the retina and cornea.

Overdose of vitamin A

The tolerable level for vitamin A, for an adult is 3,000 micrograms/day, (10,000 IU). Too much vitamin A can be harmful or fatal, resulting in what is known as hypervitaminosis A. The body converts the dimerized form, carotene, into vitamin A as it is needed; therefore high levels of carotene are not toxic compared to the ester (animal) forms (Bjelakovic *et al.*, 2007). The livers of animals from polar environments often contain amounts of vitamin A that would be toxic to humans. Hence vitamin A toxicity is typically reported in Arctic explorers and people taking large doses of synthetic vitamin A.

Effects in presence of zinc and iron

***Zinc*:** Zinc deficiency results in decreased synthesis of retinol binding protein (RBP), which transports retinol through the circulation to tissues (*e.g.*, the retina) and also protects the organism against potential toxicity of retinol. Zinc is required for the enzyme that converts retinol into retinal. At present, the health consequences of zinc deficiency on vitamin A nutritional status in humans are unclear (Brown, 2002).

***Iron*:** The combination of supplemental vitamin A and iron seems to reduce anemia more effectively than either supplemental iron or vitamin A alone (Brown, 2002). Vitamin A supplementation has beneficial effects on iron deficiency anemia and improves iron nutritional status among children and pregnant women.

As per Linus Pauling Institute's recommendation (Higdon, 2003), high potency vitamin A supplements should not be used without medical supervision due to the risk of toxicity.

Beta-carotene

Beta-carotene (β-carotene) is a member of a family of molecules known as the carotenoids. These have a basic structure made up of isoprene units. Beta-carotene is made up of eight isoprene units, which are cyclised at each end.

Functions

Beta-carotene is the most potent precursor of vitamin A, but its conversion to vitamin A in the body is limited by a feedback system. Beta carotene has two roles in the body. It can be converted into vitamin A (retinol) if the body needs more vitamin A. If the body has enough vitamin A, instead of being converted, beta carotene acts as an antioxidant which protects cells from damage caused by harmful free radicals. It is the most potent singlet oxygen quencher '*in vivo*' and the best-known and studied carotenoid due to its importance as precursor of retinol. It is found in all the cellular membranes. It exhibits strong antioxidant activity at low partial pressures of oxygen (15 torr) (Tanumihardjo, 2002). Vitamin E can protect the conjugated double bonds of β-carotene from oxidation.

Deficiency

Symptoms of a beta-carotene deficiency are similar to vitamin A deficiency: dry skin, night blindness and increased susceptibility to infection. Such deficiencies are seen especially in people lacking dietary fruits or vegetables or take supplements, because so many other foods also supply the nutrient.

Sources

Beta-carotene is the pigment that gives carrots, sweet potatoes, and other yellow vegetables their characteristic color. Plants contain other carotenoids, some of which are precursors for vitamin A (*e.g.*, alpha-carotene, beta-carotene, and beta-cryptoxanthin) (Kiefer *et al.*, 2001). Spirulina (blue-green algae) is also one of the rich sources of carotenoids.

Yellow and orange fruits, such as mangoes and papayas, orange, root vegetables such as carrots and yams are also the rich sources. Green leafy vegetables such as spinach, amaranth, colocasia and drumstick leaves contain significant amounts of carotenoids, though these pigments are masked by the green color of chlorophyll. Vietnam Gac (*Momordica cochinchinensis* spreng) and crude palm oil have by far the highest content of α-carotene of any known fruit or vegetable. However, Gac is quite rare and unknown outside its native region of SE

Asia, and unfortunately, crude palm oil is typically processed to remove the carotenoids before sale to improve the color and clarity.

RDA

No RDA has yet been established for beta-carotene since beta-carotene is converted into vitamin A in the body. The exact conversion factor varies with the circumstances; in general, 1 unit of beta-carotene in foods is thought to yield 0.25 units of vitamin A. Adults and teenagers need 6 to 15 milligrams of beta-carotene (the equivalent of 10,000 to 25,000 Units of vitamin A activity) per day (FAO-WHO rep, 1967; Rep of NAP, 2001). Children need 3 to 6 mg of beta-carotene (the equivalent of 5,000 to 10,000 Units of vitamin A activity) per day. For general health, 15 to 50 mg (25,000 to 83,000 IU) per day is recommended. The RDA for vitamin A for women who are breast-feeding increases from 800 mcg RE to 1300 mcg RE. This can be met by increasing the intake of beta carotene rich foods. Smokers should be made aware that supplemental intake of beta-carotene of 20 milligrams daily or greater were associated with a higher incidence of lung cancer in smokers.

Health disorders

A low dietary intake of carotenoids such as beta-carotene is not known to directly cause any diseases or health conditions, at least in the short term. However, long-term inadequate intake of carotenoids is associated with chronic diseases, including heart disease and various cancers (Koushik *et al.*, 2006). One important mechanism for this carotenoid-disease relationship appears to be free radicals. Research indicates that diets low in beta-carotene and carotenoids can increase the body's susceptibility to damage from free radicals. As a result, over the long term, beta-carotene deficient diets may increase tissue damage from free radical activity, and increased risk of chronic diseases like heart disease and cancers. Diets low in beta carotene may reduce the effectiveness of the immune system and lead to an increased risk of cancer and heart disease. Old persons with type 2 diabetes have shown a significant age-related decline in blood levels of carotenoids, irrespective of their dietary intake.

Overdose and toxicity

High intake of carotenoid-containing foods or supplements is not associated with any toxic side effects but the skin may turn slightly yellow-orange in color when extra large amounts are taken and will return to normal with decreased dosage (Stahl *et al.*, 1998). However, long-term use of beta-carotene supplements, especially at doses considerably above the amount necessary to supply adequate vitamin A, might slightly increase the risk of heart disease and certain forms of cancer. Beta-carotene supplementation may also decrease blood levels of lutein, another important carotenoid.

The most common side effect of excessive β-carotene consumption is carotenodermia, a harmless condition that presents as a conspicuous orange skin tint arising from deposition of the carotenoid in the outermost layer of the epidermis. Chronic, high doses of β-carotene supplements have been associated with increased rate of lung cancer among those who smoke (Tanvetyanon, 2008; Russel, 2002). Additionally, supplemental beta-carotene may increase the risk of prostate cancer. Thus moderation in use of this vitamer and avoiding inadvocate or self prescribed use without consultation with expert should be avoided.

Ascorbic Acid (Vitamin C)

Vitamin C, biochemically known as ascorbic acid, is a water-soluble vitamin. Unlike most mammals, humans lack the ability to make their own vitamin C. Therefore, we need to obtain vitamin C through our diet. Among the water-soluble vitamins, it is the most effective, least toxic antioxidant of mammalian systems and has been shown to react directly with superoxide and hydroxy radicals (Machlin and Bendich, 1987). But, in the presence of transition metals, it is known to provoke the formation of free radicals.

Functions

Vitamin C is needed for the growth and repair of tissues in all parts of the body. It is required for the synthesis of collagen, an important structural component of blood vessels, tendons, ligaments, and bone. It is essential for healing wounds, and for repairing and maintaining bones and teeth. Vitamin C also plays an important role in the synthesis of the neurotransmitter, norepinephrine. Neurotransmitters are critical to brain function and are known to affect mood. In addition, vitamin C is required for the synthesis of carnitine, a small molecule that is essential for the transport of fat to cellular organelles called mitochondria, for conversion to energy.

Vitamin C is a highly potent antioxidant. Even in small amounts, it can protect indispensable molecules in the body, such as proteins, lipids (fats), carbohydrates, and nucleic acids, DNA and RNA from damage by free radicals and reactive oxygen species that can be generated during normal metabolism as well as through exposure to toxins and pollutants (*e.g.* smoking). Vitamin C may also be able to regenerate other antioxidants such as vitamin E.

RDA

The RDA is based primarily on the prevention of deficiency disease, rather than the prevention of chronic disease and the promotion of optimum health. In the U.S., the recommended dietary allowance (RDA) for vitamin C is 60 mg daily for men and women (Carr and Frei, 1999; Food and Nutrition Board Bulletin). The RDA for Indians is 40 mg/day for sedentary adults (ICMR, 2004). Smokers are under increased oxidative stress from the toxins in cigarette smoke that deplete the blood levels of vitamin C, hence recommended intake for smokers is higher than that for nonsmokers (Bruno *et al.*, 2006). Smoking, use of oral contraceptives, the antibiotic tetracycline and barbiturates may decrease the efficacy of vitamin C.

Deficiency

Evidence suggests many people might be mildly deficient in vitamin C, although serious deficiencies may be rare in industrialized countries. Smoking cigarettes lowers the amount of vitamin C in the body, so smokers are at a higher risk of deficiency. Signs of vitamin deficiency include dry and splitting hair; gingivitis (inflammation of the gums) and bleeding gums; rough, dry, scaly skin; decreased wound-healing rate, easy bruising; nosebleeds; and a decreased ability to ward off infection. A severe form of vitamin C deficiency is known as scurvy which is a potentially fatal disease.

Scurvy: Symptoms of scurvy include bleeding and bruising easily, hair and tooth loss, joint pain and swelling. Such symptoms appear to be related to the weakening of blood vessels, connective tissue, and bone, which contain collagen (Sauberlich, 1997; Stephen, 2001). Scurvy is rare in developed countries because it can be prevented by as little as 10 mg of vitamin C daily (Weinstein, 2001).

Dietary Sources

Some excellent sources of vitamin C are gooseberries, oranges, papaya, grapefruit, cantaloupe, strawberries, kiwi, mango, broccoli, tomatoes and Brussels sprouts. Raw leafy greens (turnip greens, spinach), red and green peppers, raspberries, blueberries, cranberries, and pineapple are also rich sources of vitamin C. Vitamin C is sensitive to light, air, and heat, so the consumption of vitamin C rich sources is recommended in either raw or lightly cooked form.

Role in health disorders

Cardiovascular disease and hypertension: Vitamin C doesn't lower cholesterol levels or reduce the overall risk of heart attack, but evidence suggests that it may help protect arteries against damage. Some studies suggest that Vitamin C can slow down the progression of atherosclerosis (hardening of the arteries). It helps prevent damage to LDL ("bad") cholesterol, which then builds up as plaque in the arteries and can cause heart attack or stroke (Ye and Song, 2008, Langlois *et al.*, 2001). Other studies suggest that vitamin C may help keep arteries flexible (Cook *et al.*, 2007). People who have low levels of vitamin C may be more likely to have a heart attack, stroke all potential results of having atherosclerosis. But there is no evidence that taking vitamin C supplements will help. Population based studies suggest that people who eat foods rich in antioxidants, including vitamin C, have a lower risk of high blood pressure than people who have poorer diets. The dieticians most frequently recommend for treatment and prevention of high blood pressure, known as the DASH (Dietary Approaches to Stop Hypertension) diet, includes lots of fruits and vegetables, which are loaded with antioxidants.

Common cold: Despite the prevailing popular belief that vitamin C can cure the common cold, the scientific evidence is insufficient. Taking vitamin C supplements regularly (not just at the beginning of a cold) produces only a small reduction in the duration of a cold (Audera *et al.*, 2001).

Cataracts and age-related macular degeneration: Vitamin C (500 mg) along with zinc (80 mg), beta-carotene (15 mg), and vitamin E (400 IU) may protect the eyes against developing macular degeneration (AMD) (AREDS, 2001), the leading cause of legal blindness in people over 55 in the United States. High-dose supplementation with vitamins C and E and beta-carotene was associated with decreased incidence of age-related cataract (Taylor *et al.*, 2002; Devamanoharan *et al.*, 1991). Subnormal levels of plasma vitamin C and beta-carotene were found to be associated with higher incidence of senile cataracts among Indians (Tarwadi and Agte, 2004).

***Cancer*:** Results of many population based studies (evaluating groups of people over time) suggest that eating foods rich in vitamin C may be associated with lower rates of cancer, including skin cancer and, possibly, breast cancer. But these foods also contain many beneficial nutrients and antioxidants, not only vitamin C, so it is impossible to say for certain that vitamin C is protecting against cancer. Taking vitamin C supplements, on the other hand, did not have any helpful effect. Further, there is no evidence that taking large doses of vitamin C after diagnosed with cancer will help the treatment. More research is needed on this aspect.

***Pre-eclampsia*:** Pre-eclampsia, characterized by high blood pressure and too much protein in the urine, is a common cause of pre-term births. One of the studies suggests that taking vitamin C along with vitamin E may help prevent pre-eclampsia in women who are at high risk (Cook *et al.*, 2007).

***Hyperglycemia*:** Effect of vitamin C supplementation on blood glucose, serum lipids and serum insulin in type 2 diabetes patients were investigated in one of the studies (Afkhami, 2007). Results showed that supplemented group was benefitted and had lower blood glucose levels than the unsupplemented group. In a separate study, development and progression of long-term complications of IDDM were alleviated with supplementation of vitamin C (DCCTRG Report, 1993).

***Asthma*:** Studies are mixed when it comes to the effect of vitamin C on asthma. Some show that low levels of vitamin C are more common in people with asthma, leading some researchers to think that low levels of vitamin C might increase the risk for this condition. Other studies seem to show that vitamin C may help to reduce symptoms of exercise-induced asthma.

***Osteoarthritis*:** Vitamin C is essential for the body to make collagen, which is a part of normal cartilage. Cartilage is destroyed in osteoarthritis (OA), putting pressure on bones and joints. Yet, no evidence suggests that taking vitamin C supplements will help treat or prevent OA. What the evidence does show is that people who eat diets rich in vitamin C are less likely to be diagnosed with arthritis (Canter *et al.*, 2007).

Ascorbic acid reduces transition metals, such as cupric ions (Cu^{2+}), to cuprous (Cu^{1+}), and ferric ions (Fe^{3+}) to ferrous (Fe^{2+}) during conversion from ascorbate to dehydroxyascorbate *in vitro*. This reaction can generate superoxide and other ROS. Therefore, studies that report a antioxidant effect for vitamin C should be evaluated carefully. Nevertheless, as per the food pyramid, consuming at least five servings of fruits and vegetables daily may provide sufficient amount of vitamin C.

VITAMIN E

Naturally occurring vitamin E exists in eight different chemical forms (alpha-, beta-, gamma-, and delta-tocopherol and alpha-, beta-, gamma-, and delta-tocotrienol) that have varying levels of biological activity (Traber, 2006). Since Alpha- (or β-) tocopherol is the only form that is recognized to meet human requirements and is actively maintained in the human body; therefore, it is the form of vitamin E found in the largest quantities in blood and tissues (Traber, 2006).

Functions

Among the fat-soluble vitamins, only α-tocopherol is present in all the cellular membranes and acts as a potent peroxyl radical scavenger. Vitamin E is a fat-soluble antioxidant that stops the production of ROS formed when fat undergoes oxidation. It acts directly with oxy radicals like $O_2^{\cdot}$, ROO·, HO. and $O_2^{\cdot-}$. It helps in glutathione recycling, and maintaining reduced glutathione levels in the lens and aqueous humor (Trebor *et al.*, 2007). Being the fat-soluble vitamin, alpha-tocopherol, is uniquely suited to intercept free radicals and thus prevent a chain reaction of lipid destruction. Apart from maintaining the integrity of cell membranes throughout the body, alpha-tocopherol also protects the fats in low density lipoproteins (LDL) from oxidation.

When a molecule of alpha-tocopherol neutralizes a free radical, it is altered in such a way that its antioxidant capacity is lost. However, other antioxidants, such as vitamin C, are capable of regenerating the antioxidant capacity of alpha-tocopherol (Trebor, 2006; Sen *et al.*, 2006).

Several other functions of alpha-tocopherol have been identified that are not likely to be related to its antioxidant capacity. It is known to inhibit the activity of protein kinase C, an important cell-signaling molecule. Alpha-tocopherol appears also to affect the expression and activities of molecules and enzymes in immune and inflammatory cells. Additionally, alpha-tocopherol has been shown to inhibit platelet aggregation and to enhance vasodilation (Dietrich *et al.*, 2006; Verhagen *et al.*, 2006).

RDA

The RDA for vitamin E was previously 8 mg/day for women and 10 mg/day for men. The RDA (15 mg/day) was revised by the Food and Nutrition Board of the Institute of Medicine in 2000 (Dietrich *et al.*, 2006). Based on the results of studies done in the 1950s in men fed vitamin E deficient diets, this new recommendation was made. The breakdown of red blood cells with hydrogen peroxide known as hemolysis, was used to indicate vitamin E deficiency. Because hemolysis was reported in children with severe vitamin E deficiency, this was considered a clinically relevant test of vitamin E status.

Dietary sources

Vitamin E is found in a wide variety of foods. Major dietary sources of alpha-tocopherol include vegetable oils (olive, sunflower, and safflower oils), nuts, whole grains, and green leafy vegetables. All eight forms of vitamin E (alpha-, beta-, gamma-, and delta-tocopherols and tocotrienols) occur naturally in foods but in varying amounts. The richest sources are plant oils. Other good source is the wheat germ (found in cereals and cereal products).

Deficiency

Frank vitamin E deficiency is rare and overt deficiency symptoms have not been found in healthy people who obtain little vitamin E from their diets (NAP Report, 2000). Vitamin E deficiency has been observed in individuals with severe malnutrition, genetic defects affecting the alpha-tocopherol transfer protein, and fat malabsorption syndromes.

Because the digestive tract requires fat to absorb vitamin E, people with fat-malabsorption disorders are more likely to become deficient than people without such disorders. Peripheral neuropathy, ataxia, skeletal myopathy, retinopathy, and impairment of the immune response are the main deficiency symptoms (NAP Report, 2000; Kowdley *et al.*, 1992). People with Crohn's disease, cystic fibrosis, or an inability to secrete bile from the liver into the digestive tract, often pass greasy stools or have chronic diarrhea; as a result, they sometimes require water-soluble forms of vitamin E, (Traber, 2006; Verhagen *et al.*, 2006). Ataxia and vitamin E deficiency (AVED) is another rare, inherited disorder in which the liver's alpha-tocopherol transfer protein is defective or absent. People with AVED have such severe vitamin E deficiency that they develop nerve damage and lose the ability to walk unless they take large doses of supplemental vitamin E (Cavalier *et al.*, 1998). Children with severe vitamin E deficiency rapidly develop neurological symptoms, since the developing nervous system appears to be especially vulnerable to vitamin E deficiency. Yet, symptomatic vitamin E deficiency in healthy individuals who consume diets low in vitamin E has never been reported (Jiang *et al.*, 2001; Traber *et al.*, 2006; LPI Newsletter, 2000).

Role in health disorders

***Cataracts*:** Several studies have examined the association between vitamin E consumption and the incidence and severity of cataracts. Although results from some observational studies suggest that vitamin E may protect against cataract development, results from clinical trials do not support a preventive effect. Results of these studies are mixed: some report increased vitamin E intake protects against cataract development, while others report no association (West *et al.*, 2006). A placebo-controlled intervention trial in 4,629 men and women found that a daily antioxidant supplement containing 500 mg of vitamin C, 400 IU of synthetic vitamin E and 15 mg of beta-carotene did not affect development and progression of age-related cataracts over a 7-year period (AREDS Report, 2001). Similarly, antioxidant supplementation (500 mg of vitamin C, 400 IU alpha-tocopherol, and 15 mg of beta-carotene) did not affect progression of cataracts in a 5-year intervention trial (Gritz *et al.*, 2006). A 4-year randomized, placebo-controlled trial reported that supplements containing 500 IU/day of natural vitamin E did not reduce the incidence or progression of cataracts in older adults (McNeil *et al.*, 2004).

***Immune function*:** Alpha-tocopherol has been shown to enhance specific aspects of the immune response that appear to decline as people age. Elderly adults given 200 mg/day of synthetic alpha-tocopherol for several months displayed increased formation of antibodies in response to hepatitis B vaccine and tetanus vaccine (Meydani *et al.*, 2004). A daily supplementation with 200 IU of synthetic alpha-tocopherol for one year significantly lowered the risk of contracting upper respiratory tract infections. More research is needed to determine whether supplemental vitamin E may protect the elderly against the other infections.

***Cancer*:** The ability of alpha-tocopherol to neutralize free radicals has made it the subject of a number of cancer prevention studies. However, several large prospective studies have failed to find significant associations between alpha-tocopherol intake and the incidence of lung or breast cancer (Slatore *et al.*, 2008). One study in a cohort of 77,126 men and women reported that use of vitamin E supplements over a 10-year period increased risk of lung cancer in current smokers (Alkhenizan *et al.*, 2007). Moreover, randomized controlled trials conducted on women concluded that vitamin E supplementation was not associated with overall cancer incidence, cancer mortality, or total mortality (Lee *et al.*, 2005).

***Cardiovascular disease*:** Observational studies have suggested that supplemental alpha-tocopherol might be useful in the treatment of cardiovascular disease. A randomized, placebo-controlled intervention trial in Great Britain (the CHAOS study) found that supplementing heart disease patients with either 400 IU or 800 IU of synthetic alpha-tocopherol (equivalent to 180 mg or 360 mg of RRR-alpha-tocopherol) for an average of 18 months dramatically reduced the occurrence of nonfatal heart attacks by 77%. However, alpha-tocopherol supplementation did not significantly reduce total deaths from heart disease (Dietrich *et al.*, 2006). Supplementation of renal dialysis patients with 800 IU of natural alpha-tocopherol for an average of 1.4 years resulted in a significantly reduced risk of heart attack compared to placebo (Paolisso *et al.*, 1993). However, two other large trials in individuals with evidence of cardiovascular disease (previous heart attack, stroke, or evidence of vascular disease) found that daily supplements of 400 IU of natural alpha-tocopherol or 300 mg of synthetic alpha-tocopherol did not significantly change the risk of a subsequent heart attack or stroke (LPI Newsletter, 2000; Lee *et al.*, 2005). A trial in patients with either vascular disease or diabetes mellitus found that daily supplementation with 400 IU of natural alpha-tocopherol for an average of seven years had no effect on major cardiovascular events (myocardial infarction or stroke) or deaths; however, this study noted a slightly increased risk of heart failure in subjects taking vitamin E supplements (Lonn *et al.*, 2005). Thus, results of clinical trials using vitamin E for the treatment of heart disease have been inconsistent.

***Diabetes mellitus*:** Studies for the effect of alpha-tocopherol supplementation on blood glucose control have been contradictory. One study found a biochemical marker of oxidative stress (urinary excretion of F_2-isoprostanes) was elevated in type 2 diabetic individuals, and supplementation with 600 mg of synthetic alpha-tocopherol for 14 days reduced levels of the biomarker (Paolisso *et al.*, 1993). Some studies (Paolisso *et al.*, 1994, 1993) have shown that supplemental vitamin E improves insulin action and glucose disposal in type 2 diabetic and non-diabetic individuals, while other study has reported no improvements in glucose metabolism of type 2 diabetics (River *et al.*, 1995). One study reported that supplementing type 1 diabetics with only 100 IU/day of synthetic alpha-tocopherol for one month significantly improved both glycosylated hemoglobin and triglyceride levels (Jain *et al.*, 1996) though research reveals its supplementation to be beneficial in treatment for type 1 or type 2 diabetes, evidence from well-controlled clinical trials is underscored.

A study analyzed 50 Wistar rats for 90 days and divided them into five groups of 10 rats. One group was given standard rat diet and the others received the methionine and choline deficient diet. One received saline 0.9% and the others received metformin, vitamin E or simvastatin. Groups that received standard rat diet and methionine and choline deficient with vitamin E presented significantly lower rates of lipid peroxides. The presence of fibrosis was significantly smaller in the group receiving vitamin E indicating that the vitamin reduced the liver oxidative stress, as well as the fibrosis development.

The effects of alpha-tocopherol supplementation on the cardiopulmonary fitness in endurance athletes (cyclists) and non-athletes were investigated in one study wherein various physiological parameters like heart rate, blood pressure, respiratory rate for assessing cardiopulmonary fitness were recorded before and after supplementation of vitamin E in athletes, and were compared with placebo group before and after supplementation of placebo and also with non-athletes. The results indicated that alpha-tocopherol supplementation did not contribute significantly to improve the cardiopulmonary fitness of endurance athletes. Thus α-tocopherol looks to be a promising dietary supplement for maintenance of health and prevention of diseases.

An Overview of Vitamins (Tables 2.1-2.15)

Some recent research related to thiamin

Arsenic exposure is a major public health problem in Bangladesh, where nearly 77 million people have been chronically exposed to arsenic through the consumption of naturally contaminated groundwater. Increasing dietary intakes of thiamin, niacin, pantothenic acid, and pyridoxine were found to significantly increase urinary total arsenic excretion, adjusted for daily arsenic intake from drinking water and other potential confounders (Argos *et al.,* 2010). The case of a 63-year-old woman with thiamine deficiency who showed auditory hallucinations, a delusion of persecution, catatonic stupor, and catalepsy but no neurological symptoms including oculomotor or gait disturbance indicates that the possibility of thiamine deficiency should be considered in cases of psychosis without neurological disturbance and high-intensity T2 MRI lesions (Sasaki *et al.*, 2010).

Table 2.1: Thiamin at glance

Name	*Biological function*	*Preventive role in diseases*	*Toxic effects*	*RDA*
Thiamin	Thiamin pyrophosphate (TPP) is a required coenzyme for Pyruvate dehydrogenase,-ketoglutarate dehydrogenase, and branched chain ketoacid (BCKA) dehydrogenase which play critical roles in the production of energy from food. Transketolase (TPP) catalyzes the pentose phosphate pathway. TTP activates membrane ion channels, possibly by phosphorylation.	Thiamin deficiency results in peripheral neuropathy, burning feet syndrome, abnormal reflexes, diminished sensation and weakness in legs and arms. Muscle pain and tenderness and difficulty rising from a squatting position. Severely thiamin deficient individuals may experience seizures. Enlargement of the heart, severe swelling, difficulty breathing, and congestive heart failure confused apathetic state or a profound memory disorder.	No known toxic effects from the consumption of excess thiamin in food or through long-term oral supplementation (up to 200 mg/ day).	Infants: 200–300 µg, Children 500–900 µg, Adolescents: 1200 µg, Adults: 1200 µg, Pregnancy: 1400 µg, Lactation: 1400 µg, Indian men: 1.2 mg Indian women: 1.1 mg.

Some recent research related to riboflavin

Smoking lowered circulating concentrations of folate, PLP, and riboflavin, but concentrations increased significantly after a few days of smoking cessation (Ulvik *et al.*, 2010). Riboflavin is immune protective in humans, and this may reflect the role of the B group vitamins in cellular energy restoration after UV exposure (Damian *et al.*, 2010).

Table 2.2: Riboflavin at glance

Name	*Biological function*	*Preventive role in diseases*	*Toxic effects*	*RDA*
Riboflavin	Flavin coenzymes participate in carbohydrates, fats, and protein metabolism. FAD in conjunction with cytochrome P-450 participates in metabolism of drugs and toxins. FAD plays a major role in protecting organisms from reactive oxygen species, such as hydroperoxides and the oxidation of hypoxanthine and xanthine to uric acid the most effective water-soluble antioxidants in the blood.	Sore throat, redness and swelling of the lining of the mouth, tongue, and throat, cracks or sores on the outsides of the lips, at the corners of the mouth, scaly skin, formation of blood vessels in the clear covering of the eye, and decreased red blood cell count. Riboflavin deficiency alters iron metabolism, increases risk preeclampsia in pregnant women.	No toxic or adverse effects of high riboflavin intake in humans are known.	Infants: 65 µg/kg, Children: 700–1200 µg, Adolescents: 1200–1600 µg, Adults: 1400–1900 µg, Pregnancy: 1800 µg, Lactation: 1600 µg, Indian men: 1.4 mg, Indian women: 1.3 mg.

Some recent research related to nicotinic acid

Niacin treatment caused a moderate increase in the ability of HDL to promote net cholesterol efflux, whereas inhibition of cholesteryl ester transfer protein via anacetrapib led to a more dramatic increase in association with enhanced particle functionality at higher HDL concentrations. All HDLs exhibited potent ability to suppress macrophage toll-like receptor 4-mediated inflammatory responses, in a process partly dependent on cholesterol efflux (Yvan-Charvet *et al.*, 2010). Niacin has been used for decades to treat dyslipidaemic disorders. Niacin is the most effective agent currently available for increasing levels of high-density lipoprotein. Moreover, significant improvements in cardiovascular outcomes in niacin treated patients have been demonstrated. Since tolerability concerns, particularly flushing, have limited its use, ER niacin, a prolonged-release formulation of niacin, has been developed with similar efficacy but a superior tolerability profile compared to immediate-release formulations (Benhalima and Muls, 2010).

Table 2.3: Nicotinic acid at glance

Name	*Biological function*	*Preventive role in diseases*	*Toxic effects*	*RDA*
Nicotinic acid	200 enzymes require the niacin coenzymes, NAD and NADP for redox reactions, catabolism of carbohydrates, fats, proteins, and alcohol to produce energy anabolic reactions, in synthesis of fatty acids and cholesterol. Cell signaling and differentiation.	The symptoms of pellagra: dermatitis, diarrhea, dementia, and death. In the skin, a thick, scaly, darkly pigmented rash develops in areas exposed to sunlight. Preventive role in cancer, insulin dependant diabetes, coronary heart disease and acquired immunodeficiency syndrome (AIDS).	Hepatotoxicity (liver cell damage), including elevated liver enzymes and jaundice, has been observed at intakes 750 mg nicotinic acid/day for less than 3 months. UL for niacin 30 mg.	Infants: 2–4 mg Children: 6–12 mg, Adolescents: 16 mg, Adults: 16 mg, Pregnancy: 18 mg, Lactation: 17 mg Indian adults: 16 mg.

Some recent research related to folic acid

A recent study (Hoch *et al.*, 2010) has demonstrated that brachial artery flow-mediated dilation (FMD), an indicator of vascular endothelial function, improves in amenorrheic female runners after short-term supplementation with folic acid. Among patients with diabetic nephropathy, high doses of B vitamins; folic acid, vitamin B(6), and vitamin B(12)compared with placebo resulted in a greater decrease in GFR and an increase in vascular events (House *et al.*, 2010). Another study revealed serious deficiencies in the intakes of several vitamins and essential nutrients (Xia *et al.*, 2010). A meta-analysis of 12 trials of multiple micronutrient supplementation compared with iron-folic acid reveals an overall 11% reduction in low birth weight but no effect on preterm birth and perinatal or neonatal survival. Currently, data are unconvincing for replacing supplementation of antenatal iron-folic acid with multiple micronutrients (Christian, 2010).

Table 2.4: Folic acid at glance

Name	*Biological function*	*Preventive role in diseases*	*Toxic effects*	*RDA*
Folic acid	One-carbon metabolism, nucleic acid metabolism, amino acid metabolism, homocysteine in blood is regulated by three vitamins: folic acid, vitamin B-12, and vitamin B-6.	Pregnancy complications: Neural tube defects Alzheimer's disease, Breast cancer, Colorectal cancer Cardiovascular diseases (heart disease, stroke, and peripheral vascular diseases).	Food folic acid safe. Children: 400 µg, Adolescents: 800 µg, Adults: 1000 µg.	Infants: 80 µg, Children: 150–300 µg, Adolescents: 400 µg, Adults: 400 µg, Pregnancy: 600 µg, Lactation: 500 µg, Indian adults: 100 µg.

Some recent research related to pyridoxine

Pyridoxin-dependent seizures are inherited in an autosomal recessive manner and characterized by intractable seizures that are not controlled with anticonvulsants but that respond to large daily supplements of pyridoxin (Gospe, 2009). Primary hyperoxaluria type 1 (PH1) is caused by a deficiency of the liver peroxisomal enzyme alanine: glyoxylate-aminotransferase. Prevention of primary manifestation include maintenance of high fluid intake; pyridoxine supplements for those who are pyridoxine responsive (Coulter-Mackie *et al.*, 2009). Endothelial cells exposed to 0.5 mM hydrogen peroxide for 2 hours increased the superoxide anion and lipid peroxide levels as biomarkers of oxidative stress. Results indicate that pyridoxamine, pyridoxine, and pyridoxal phosphate acted as antioxidants and reduced the superoxide and lipid peroxides induced by hydrogen peroxide, but did not protect the cells from the effects directly related to hydrogen peroxide itself (Mahfouz *et al.*, 2009).

Table 2.5: Pyridoxin at glance

Name	*Biological function*	*Preventive role in diseases*	*Toxic effects*	*RDA*
Pyridoxin	Coenzyme, PLP plays a vital role in: release of glucose stored as glycogen, generation of glucose from amino acids, synthesis of dopamine, norepinephrine and gamma-aminobutyric acid (GABA), synthesis of heme, serotonin, and niacin from tryptophan. The binding of PLP to steroid receptors for estrogen, progesterone, testosterone, and other steroid hormones may have implications for breast cancer and prostate cancer, involved in the synthesis of nucleic acids.	Abnormal EEG (electro-encephalogram) patterns neurologic symptoms noted in severe vitamin B-6 deficiency include irritability, depression, and confusion, inflammation of the tongue, sores or ulcers of the mouth, and ulcers of the skin at the corners of the mouth.	Sensory neuropathy typically develops at doses of pyridoxine in excess of 1,000 mg per day.	Men and women 19–50 y: 1.3 mg, Men 51 y and older: 1.7 mg, Women 51 y and older: 1.5 mg, Indian adults: 2 mg.

Some recent research related to vitamin B12

Caution has been indicated before widespread folic acid fortification of food, without addressing the issue of concurrent B12 deficiency in treatment of Neural tube defects (NTDs) (Godbole *et al.,* 2009). Hyperhomocysteinemia is generally acknowledged as a treatable risk factor for atherothrombotic diseases. Because of the low cost and safety of the therapy, the American Heart and Stroke Association advises to treat patients with a stroke and hyperhomocysteinemia daily with 0.4 mg folic acid, 2.4 mcg vitamin B12 and 1.7 mg vitamin B6 (Terwecoren *et al.*, 2009). Stroke is a leading cause of death in developed countries. Poor dietary intake of folate, vitamin B6 and vitamin B12 are associated with increased risk of stroke (Sánchez-Moreno *et al.,* 2009).

Table 2.6: Vitamin B12 at glance

Name	*Biological function*	*Preventive role in diseases*	*Toxic effects*	*RDA*
Cyano-cobal-amin (B12)	Cofactor for methionine synthase: required for the synthesis of methionine, from homocysteine used in many biological methylation reactions, (may be important in cancer prevention). Cofactor for L-methyl-malonyl-CoA mutase: plays an important role in the production of energy from fats and proteins. Succinyl CoA is also required for the synthesis of hemoglobin.	Pernicious anemia, Megaloblastic anemia, Neurologic symptoms: numb-ness and tingling of the arms/legs, difficulty in walking, memory loss, disorientation and dementia, with or without mood changes. Gastroin-testinal symptoms: A sore tongue, appetite loss, and constipation cardiovascular diseases risk.	Safe upto 1000 µg.	Adults and young: 2.4 µg Pregnancy: 2.6 µg/day Indian adults and young: 1 µg.

Some recent research related to CoQ_{10}

Studies in apolipoprotein E-deficient mice, an animal model of atherosclerosis, found that coenzyme Q_{10} supplementation with supra-pharmacological amounts of coenzyme Q_{10} significantly inhibited the formation of free radicals (Sohal *et al.*, 2006). Co-Q_{10} levels were measured annually in a prospective cohort study of 381 children with Cystic Fibrosis (CF) (Laguna *et al.*, 2008). Of the 381 initial total serum Co-Q_{10} measurements, 188 were in the deficient range. Low Co-Q_{10} was significantly more prevalent in patients with pancreatic insufficiency (PI) (55%) compared with patients with pancreatic sufficiency (PS) (3%); Low Co-Q_{10} levels were related to other markers of nutritional status, including total lipids, beta-carotene, and alpha tocopherol. The recent history of clinical trials of dichloro-acetate, arginine, coenzyme Q_{10}, idebenone, and exercise in both primary (congenital) disorders and secondary (degenerative) disorders was reviewed (Kerr, 2010). A controlled clinical trial is now underway to exmine its effects to prevent the progression of Parkinson disease. CoQ_{10} is now used as a nutritional supplement because of its antioxidant properties and is beneficial in the treatment of several human diseases when administered orally (Jeya *et al.*, 2010).

Table 2.7: Coenzyme Q_{10} at glance

Name	*Biological function*	*Preventive role in diseases*	*Toxic effects*	*RDA*
Coenzyme Q_{10}	Production of a high-energy compound called ATP.	Cardiomyopathy (heart muscle disease) and congestive heart failure protects against oxidation of LDLs (the bad cholesterol that gets even more atherogenic with oxidative stress), in hyperlipidemic patients and hypertension and may also help to slow the aging process	No adverse effects up to 100 mg/day.	30–45 mg.

Some recent research related to vitamin (B5)

The physiological roles of pantothenic acid (PaA) on testicular function, in particular, testicular endocrinology and sperm mortility, were investigated in rats. Male rats at 3 weeks of age were fed a PaA-free diet or a 0.0016% PaA diet (control) for 7 weeks. The relative weights of the testes were significantly higher in the PaA-deficient group compared with the control group. Several parameters of sperm motility were significantly reduced in the PaA-deficient group compared with the control group. Thus, PaA is an essential factor in testicular endocrinology and sperm motility in male rats (Yamamoto *et al.*, 2009).

Pantethine, the stable disulfide form of pantetheine, is the major precursor of coenzyme A, which plays a central role in the metabolism of lipids and carbohydrates. This molecule is a well-tolerated therapeutic agent; the frequency of its side-effect is very low and mild. Based on the preclinical and clinical data, it could be recommended using this

Table 2.8: Pantothenic acid at glance

Name	*Biological function*	*Toxic effects*	*RDA*
Pantothenic acid Calcium pantothenate and Panthenol (B5)	Utilization of other nutrients; Maintaining normal growth and development of the nervous system; Metabolism of fat and sugars.	Very large doses have been known to produce lack of co-ordination in movement and impairment of sensation.	RDA for adults is 7 mg.

compound as adjuvant therapy. Pantethine has beneficial effects in vascular disease, it is able to decrease the hyperlipidaemia, moderate the platelet function and prevent the lipid-peroxidation. Moreover its neuro-endocrinological regulating role, its good influence on cataract and cystinosis are also proved (Horwath and Vecsei, 2009).

Some recent research related to Biotin

Animal studies have indicated few, if any, effects due to toxic doses of biotin. This may provide evidence that both animals and humans could tolerate doses of at least an order of magnitude greater than each of their nutritional requirements. There are no reported cases of adverse effects from receiving high doses of the vitamin, particularly when used in the treatment of metabolic disorders causing sebhorrheic dermatitis in infants (Murray *et al.*, 1997; Combs and Gerald, 1998).

Children with a rare inherited metabolic disorder called phenylketonuria (PKU; in which one is unable to break down the amino acid phenylalanine) often develop skin conditions such as eczema and seborrheic dermatitis in areas of the body other than the scalp. The scaly skin changes that occur in people with PKU may be related to poor ability to use biotin. Increasing dietary biotin has been known to improve seborrheic dermatitis in these cases. Diabetics may also benefit from biotin supplementation. In both insulin-dependent and non-insulin-dependent diabetes, supplementation with biotin can improve blood sugar control and help lower fasting blood glucose levels, in some studies the reduction in fasting glucose exceeded 50 percent. Biotin can also play a role in preventing the neuropathy often associated with diabetes, reducing both the numbness and tingling associated with poor glucose control (Higdon, 2003).

Table 2.9: Biotin at glance

Name	*Biological function*	*Preventive role in diseases*	*Toxic effects*	*RDA*
Biotin	It is essential for the metabolism of fats and the synthesis of ascorbic acid. It maintains a healthy skin and helps to prevent baldness and hair from turning grey.	Needed during rapid growth periods in glucose metabolism.	Not toxic.	RDA for adults is 100 mg.

Some recent research related to Choline

Women having diets richer in choline may have a lower risk for breast cancer (Xu *et al.*, 2008, 2009) but other studies found no association (Cho *et al.*, 2007, 2010). A small study found that choline supplements reduced symptoms of allergic rhinitis (Das *et al.*, 2005). There is some evidence that choline is anti-inflammatory. In one study, higher dietary intake of choline was associated with lower levels of inflammatory markers (Panagiotakos *et al.*, 2008).

Despite its importance in the central nervous system as a precursor for acetylcholine and membrane phosphatidylcholine, the role of choline in mental illness has been little studied. In a large population-based study, blood levels of choline were inversely correlated with anxiety symptoms in subjects aged 46–49 and 70–74 years. However, there was no correlation between depression and choline level in this study (Bjelland *et al.*, 2009).

Table 2.10: Choline at glance

Name	*Biological function*	*Preventive role in diseases*	*Toxic effects*	*RDA*
Choline (cofactor of the B vitamins).	Essential for growth; Involved in fat transport, carbohydrate and protein metabolism. It is crucial for normal brain functioning and memory.	Aids in the treatment of Alzheimer's disease and helps to remove drugs and poisons from our body.	No known toxicity.	No RDA but the average adult diet contains between 500 milligrams to 900 milligrams a day.

Some recent research related to ascorbic acid

The antioxidant vitamins C and E appear to be particularly beneficial for combating age-related oxidative stress when administered in combination for their potential to protect against age-related cognitive decline (Brown *et al.*, 2010). Studies were identified by performing an extensive search using BIOSIS (1986–2007), EMBASE (1986–2007), Medline (1986–2007), and the Cochrane database. Established preeclampsia is associated with increased concentrations of oxidative stress markers including lipid peroxidation products, and a reduction in antioxidant concentrations (vitamin C) (Gupta *et al.*, 2009). Nutritional supplements that might help prevent gallstones include vitamin C, soy lecithin, and iron (Gaby, 2009).

Table 2.11: Vitamin C at glance

Name	***Biological function***	***Preventive role in diseases***	***Toxic effects***	***RDA***
Vitamin C (Ascorbic acid).	Synthesis of collagen, component of blood vessels, tendons, ligaments, and bone, role in the synthesis of the neurotransmitter, norepinephrine, carnitine, essential for the transport of fat to mitochondria, involved in the metabolism of cholesterol to bile acids, a highly effective antioxidant and protects proteins, lipids (fats), carbohydrates, and nucleic acids from damage by free radicals generated during normal metabolism, exposure to toxins and pollutants.	Scurvy, Cardio-vascular diseases (heart disease and stroke), cancer, cataract, diabetes, common cold, lead toxicity.	UL for synthetic ascorbic acid; Children: 400–1200 mg, Adolescents: 800 mg, Adults: 2000 mg.	Infants and children: 15–45 mg, Adolescents: 75 mg, Adults: 90 mg, Pregnancy: 85 mg, Lactation: 115 mg, Indian adults: 40 mg.

Some recent research related to vitamin A

Vitamin A regulates germ cell differentiation and may lead to the generation of both, the cycle of the seminiferous epithelium and the spermatogenic wave (Hogarth and Griswold, 2010). A meta-analysis of the studies found that measles vaccine and vitamin A treatment are effective interventions to prevent measles mortality in children (Sudfeld *et al.*, 2010). Vitamin A supplementation given alone or in combination with iodised salt can have a beneficial impact on thyroid function and thyroid size (Hess, 2010). Ingestion of beta-carotene from foods, along with a diet rich in fruits and vegetables, has a protective role against lung disease (Cranganu and Camporeale, 2009).

Retinoic acid, derived from vitamin A, has been shown to have roles as an antioxidant and in cellular differentiation. Recent compelling evidence indicates a role of retinoic acid in cognitive activities and anti-amyloidogenic properties. The actions of retinoic acid indicate that it may have therapeutic properties ideally served for the treatment of neurodegenerative diseases such as Alzheimer's disease (Lee *et al.*, 2009).

Table 2.12: Vitamin A at glance

Name	*Biological function*	*Preventive role in diseases*	*Toxic effects*	*RDA*
Vitamin A (Retinol).	Plays role in vision cellular differentiation, immunity, growth and development and RBC production. Helps iron absorption.	Impaired dark adaptation, known as night blindness, changes in the conjunctiva (corner of the eye) called Bitot's spots. Severe or prolonged vitamin A deficiency causes xeropthalmia, increased morbidity and mortality due to infectious diseases and cancer.	Hypervitaminosis A may result in liver damage, hemorrhage, and coma. Upper level (UL) of vitamin A intake for adults at 3,000 mcg (10,000 IU)/day of preformed vitamin A.	Infants: 400 µg, Children: 300–600 µg, Adolescents: 900 µg, Men/women: 900 µg, Pregnancy: 770 µg, Lactation: 1200 µg, Indian adults: 600 µg.

Some recent research related to vitamin D

A role for supplements, including vitamin D, folate, and vitamin B6, remains uncertain, calcium supplementation is likely to be at least modestly beneficial in colorectal cancer (Chan and Giovannucci, 2010). Vitamin D and calcium may affect the cardiovascular system independently and interactively (Wang *et al.*, 2010). Prospective epidemiological studies supported by strong mechanistic evidence

Table 2.13: Vitamin D at glance

Name	*Biological function*	*Preventive role in diseases*	*Toxic effects*	*RDA*
Vitamin D	Maintenance of blood calcium levels within a narrow range, for normal functioning of the nervous system, for bone growth, and maintenance of bone density	Osteoporosis, cancer, Insulin-dependent diabetes mellitus (IDDM), multiple sclerosis (MS), and rheumatoid arthritis	Pharmacologic doses of 10, 000 to 50,000 IU/day (250 to 1250 mcg/day), loss of appetite, nausea, vomiting, excessive thirst, excessive urination, severe itching, muscular weakness, joint pain, and ultimately disorientation, coma, and death.	Men and women 19–50 yrs: 5 µg or 200 IU; Men and women 51–70 yrs: 10 µg or 400 IU; Men and women > 70 yrs: 15 µg or 600 IU

suggest a reduction of cardiovascular disease (incident hypertension and cardiovascular mortality) and colorectal cancer, extending to weaker evidence on immune-modulatory and anti-inflammatory benefits of vitamin D (Bischoff-Ferrari, 2010). The effect of vitamin D on the immune system is particularly relevant to the dermatologist in that it has implications for atopic dermatitis, psoriasis, and skin cancer (Miller and Gallo, 2010).

Some recent research related to vitamin E

In one of the studies by Salobir *et al.* (2010), oxidative stress was induced by high intake of polyunsaturated fatty acids (PUFAs) in pigs, as a model for humans. Twenty-four growing pigs were divided into four groups that received isocaloric daily rations *i.e.* linseed oil, linseed oil and black currant juice or linseed oil and vitamin E. In comparison with the Oil group, vitamin E supplementation significantly lowered plasma malondialdehyde (MDA) and the 24 h urine MDA excretion rate, and reduced the degree of DNA damage in leukocytes to the level of the control group.

To examine if vitamin E has any effect on the hemopoietic system in hypercholesterolemia, blood samples were collected before and at various intervals during a high cholesterol diet (0.25% cholesterol) for 2 and 4 months, and while on high cholesterol diet with vitamin E (2

Table 2.14: Vitamin E at glance

Name	*Biological function*	*Preventive role in diseases*	*Toxic effects*	*RDA*
Vitamin E (Tocopherol) Vitamin E is the term used for eight naturally occurring, fat-soluble nutrients called tocopherols-alpha, beta, gamma, delta, epsilon, zeta, eta and theta.	Fat-soluble antioxidant and prevents the potentially harmful oxidation of fat and enhances the functioning of vitamin A. It is an antipollutant for the lungs. It helps the healing of scar tissue when taken internally and also when applied externally.	Vitamin E deficiency may cause anemia, as a result of red blood cell destruction and neurological dysfunction, myopathies, and diminished erythrocyte life span.	Generally non-toxic but some evidence suggests that large intakes may cause increased levels of blood cholesterol and lipids.	RDA for adults is 10 IU.

months) following a high cholesterol diet (2 months). The hypercholesterolemia decreased RBC count, hematocrit and hemoglobin, increased mean corpuscular volume, red blood cell distribution width, mean corpuscular hemoglobin but had no effect on WBC and platelet counts, and mean platelet volume. Thus, hypercholesterolemia of short duration has adverse effects on certain elements of the hemopoietic system. Vitamin E did not affect any of the parameters of the hemopoietic system (Prasad, 2010).

Some recent research related to vitamin K

A high intake of phylloquinone may favorably affect Metabolic syndrome (MetS) or its components, probably through an overall more heart-healthy dietary pattern (Pan and Jackson, 2009). In a multivariate model adjusting for diabetes risk factors and dietary factors, phylloquinone intake tended to be associated ($p = 0.08$) with a reduced risk of type 2 diabetes with a hazard ratio of 0.81 (95%-CI: 0.66–0.99) for the highest versus the lowest quartile (Beulens *et al.*, 2010).

Anticarcinogenic activities of vitamin K have been observed in animal and cell studies. Dietary intake of menaquinones was non significantly inversely associated with overall cancer incidence (HR for the highest compared with the lowest quartile: 0.86; 95% CI: 0.73, 1.01; P for trend = 0.08), and the association was stronger for cancer mortality (HR: 0.72; 95% CI: 0.53, 0.98; P for trend = 0.03). Cancer risk reduction with increasing intake of menaquinones was more pronounced in men than in women, mainly driven by significant inverse associations with prostate (P for trend = 0.03) and lung (P for trend = 0.002) cancer (Nimptsch *et al.*, 2010).

Table 2.15: Vitamin K at glance

Name	*Biological function*	*Preventive role in diseases*	*Toxic effects*	*RDA*
Vitamin K Phylloquinone (K1) menaquinone-n (MK-n or K2)	Blood clotting, Bone mineralization, Cell proliferation.	Osteoporosis, Vascular calcification, Cardiovascular disease.	K1 non toxic, K2 interferes with function of glutathione, induce liver damage, anemia.	Men 19 y and older: 120 µg; women 19 y and older: 90 µg.

Thus, Vitamins the essential ingredients of our diet are present in small amounts but play a wide variety of vital functions for human body. Recent research has come out with many new biological functions and protective roles of vitamins beyond their classical functions of preventing deficiency symptoms. This is particularly true for Vitamin A,C and E.

REFERENCES

Afkhami-Ardekani M, and Shojaoddiny-Ardekani A 2007. Effect of vitamin C on blood glucose, serum lipids and serum insulin in type 2 diabetes patients. *Ind. J. Med. Res.* 126(5): 471–4.

Alkhenizan A, and Hafez K 2007. The role of vitamin E in the prevention of cancer: a meta-analysis of randomized controlled trials. *Ann Saudi Med.* 27(6): 409–414.

AREDS Report No. 9. 2001. A randomized, placebo-controlled, clinical trial of high-dose supplementation with vitamins C and E and beta carotene for age-related cataract and vision loss: *Arch. Ophthalmol.* 119(10): 1439–1452.

Argos M, Rathouz PJ, Pierce BL, *et al.* 2010. Dietary B vitamin intakes and urinary total arsenic concentration in the health effects of arsenic longitudinal study (HEALS) cohort, Bangladesh. *Eur. J. Nutr.* (Epub ahead of print).

Audera C, Patulny RV, Sander BH, and Douglas RM 2001. Mega-dose vitamin C in treatment of the common cold: a randomised controlled trial. *Med. J. Aust.* 175(7): 359–362.

Benhalima K, and Muls E Niacin 2010. An old drug with new perspectives for the management of dyslipidaemia. *Acta. Clin. Belg.* 65(1): 23–8.

Beulens JW, Van der A, Grobbee DE *et al.* 2010. Dietary phylloquinone and menaquinones intake and risk of type 2 diabetes. *Diabetes Care.* (Epub ahead of print).

Bischoff-Ferrari H 2010. Health effects of vitamin D. *Dermatol Ther.* 23(1): 23–30.

Bjelakovic *et al.* 2007. Mortality in randomized trials of antioxidant supplements for primary and secondary prevention: Systematic review and meta-analysis. *JAMA* 297: 842.

Bjelland I, Tell GS, Vollset SE, Konstantinova S, and Ueland PM 2009. Choline in anxiety and depression: the Hordaland Health Study. *Am. J. Clin. Nutr.* 90(4): 1056–60.

Brown JE, 2002. Vitamins and your health. *Nutrition Now* 3rd Ed. pp. 20–1 to 20–20.

Brown LA, Riby LM, and Reay JL 2010. Supplementing cognitive aging: a selective review of the effects of *Ginkgo biloba* and a number of everyday nutritional substances. *Exp. Aging. Res.* 36(1): 105–22.

Bruno RS, Leonard SW, Atkinson J, *et al.* 2006. Faster plasma vitamin E disappearance in smokers is normalized by vitamin C supplementation. *Free Rad. Biol. Med.* 40(4): 689–697.

Canter PH, Wider B, and Ernst E 2007. The antioxidant vitamins A, C, E and selenium in the treatment of arthritis: a systematic review of randomized clinical trials. *Rheumatology* 46(8): 1223–33.

Carr AC, and Frei B 1999. Toward a new recommended dietary allowance for vitamin C based on antioxidant and health effects in humans. *Am. J. Clin. Nutr.* 69(6): 1086–1107.

Cavalier L, Ouahchi K, Kayden H, Donato S, Reutenaucer L, Mandel JL, *et al.* 1998. Ataxia with isolated vitamin E deficiency: heterogeneity of mutations and phenotypic variability in a large number of families. *Am. J. Hum. Genet.* 62: 301–10.

Chan AT, and Giovannucci EL 2010. Primary prevention of colorectal cancer. *Gastroenterology* 138(6): 2029–2043.e10.

Cho E, Holmes M, Hankinson SE, and Willett WC 2007. Nutrients involved in one-carbon metabolism and risk of breast cancer among premenopausal women. *Cancer Epidemiology, Biomarkers & Prevention* 16(12): 2787–90.

Cho E, Holmes MD, Hankinson SE, and Willett WC 2010. Choline and betaine intake and risk of breast cancer among post-menopausal women. *Br J. Cancer* 102(3): 489–94.

Christian P, 2010. Micronutrients, Birth Weight, and Survival. *Annu Rev. Nutr.* (Epub ahead of print).

Combs Gerald F Jr 1998. The Vitamins: Fundamental Aspects in Nutrition and Health. Ithaca: Elsevier Academic Press. ISBN 0121834921. p. 360.

Cook NR, Albert CM, Gaziano JM, *et al.* 2007. A randomized factorial trial of vitamins C and E and beta carotene in secondary prevention of cardiovascular events in women: results from the Women's Antioxidant Cardiovascular Study. *Arch. Intern. Med.* 167(15): 1610–8.

Coulter-Mackie MB, White CT, Hurley RM, *et al.* 2002. Primary Hyperoxaluria Type 1. (updated 2009 Aug. 11).

Cranganu A, and Camporeale J 2009. Nutrition aspects of lung cancer. *Nutr. Clin. Pract.* 24(6): 688–700.

Damian DL, Matthews YJ, and Halliday GM 2010. Topical riboflavin attenuates ultraviolet B- and ultraviolet A-induced immunosuppression in humans. *Photodermatol Photoimmunol Photomed.* 26(2): 66–9.

Das S, Gupta K, Gupta A, and Gaur S 2005. Comparison of the efficacy of inhaled budesonide and oral choline in patients with allergic rhinitis. *Saudi Medical Journal* 26(3): 421–4.

DCCTRG report 1993. Effect of intensive research on development and progression of long-term complications of IDDM. *N. Eng. J. Med.* 329: 977–986.

Devamanoharan PS, Henein M, Morris S, *et al.* 1991. Prevention of selenite cataract by vitamin C. *Exp. Eye Res.* 52(5): 563–568.

Dietary Reference Intakes for Vitamin A, Vitamin K, Arsenic, Boron, Chromium, Copper, Iodine, Iron, Manganese, Molybdenum, Nickel, Silicon, Vanadium and Zinc. Washington, DC: National Academy Press. 2001.

Dietrich M, Traber MG, Jacques PF, *et al.* 2006. Does γ-tocopherol play a role in the primary prevention of heart disease and cancer? A review. *Am J. Coll. Nutr.* 25: 292–9.

Food and Agriculture Organization/World Health Organization. Requirement of Vitamin A, Thiamine, Riboflavin and Niacin. 1967; FAO Food and Nutrition Series B. Rome.

Food and Nutrition Board, Institute of Medicine 2000. Vitamin C. Dietary Reference Intakes for Vitamin C, Vitamin E, Selenium, and Carotenoids. Washington DC: National Academy Press. pp. 95–185.

Gaby AR 2009. Nutritional approaches to prevention and treatment of gallstones. *Altern. Med. Rev.* 14(3): 258–67.

Godbole K, Deshmukh U, and Yajnik C 2009. Nutrigenetic determinants of neural tube defects in India. *Indian Pediatr.* 46(6): 467–75.

Gospe SM Jr. 2001. Pyridoxine-Dependent Seizures. *In:* Pagon *et al.* Gene Reviews Seattle (WA): Univ. Washington 1993-2001. (updated 2009 Nov. 10).

Gritz DC, Srinivasan M, Smith SD, *et al.* 2006. The Antioxidants in prevention of cataracts study: effects of antioxidant supplements on cataract progression in South India. *Br. J. Ophthalmol.* 90(7): 847–851.

Gropper S, Smith J, and Groff J 2009. Advanced Nutrition and Human Metabolism 5th Edition pp. 373–1182.

Gupta S, Aziz N, Sekhon L, *et al.* 2009. Lipid peroxidation and antioxidant status in preeclampsia: a systematic review. *Obstet Gynecol Surv.* 64(11): 750–9.

Hess SY 2010. The impact of common micronutrient deficiencies on iodine and thyroid metabolism: the evidence from human studies. *Best. Pract. Res. Clin. Endocrinol Metab.* 24(1): 117–32.

Higdon Jane 2003. Biotin. An evidence-based approach to vitamins and minerals. Thieme. ISBN 9781588901248.

Higdon, Jane. Vitamin A; Linus Pauling Institute's Micronutrient Information Center.

Hoch AZ, Lynch SL, Jurva JW, *et al.* 2010. Folic acid supplementation improves vascular function in amenorrheic runners. *Clin. J. Sport. Med.* 20(3): 205–10.

Hogarth CA, and Griswold MD 2010. The key role of vitamin A in spermatogenesis. *J. Clin. Invest.* 120(4): 956–62.

Horváth Z, and Vécsei L 2009. Current medical aspects of pantethine. *Ideggyogy Sz.* 62(7–8): 220–9.

House AA, Eliasziw M, Cattran DC, *et al.* 2010. Effect of B-vitamin therapy on progression of diabetic nephropathy: a randomized controlled trial. *JAMA.* 303(16): 1603–9.

Institute of Medicine. Food and Nutrition Board 2000. Dietary Reference Intakes: Vitamin C, Vitamin E, Selenium, and Carotenoids. Washington, DC: National Academy Press, 2000.

Jain SK, McVie R, Jaramillo JJ, Palmer M, and Smith T 1996. Effect of modest vitamin E supplementation on blood glycated hemoglobin and triglyceride levels and red cell indices in type I diabetic patients. *J. Am. Coll. Nutr.* 15(5): 458–461.

Jeya M, Moon HJ, Lee JL, Kim IW, and Lee JK 2010. Current state of coenzyme Q(10) production and its applications. *Appl. Microbiol. Biotechnol.* 85(6): 1653–63.

Jiang Q, Christen S, Shigenaga MK, and Ames BN 2001. γ-tocopherol, the major form of vitamin E in the US diet, deserves more attention. *Am. J. Clin. Nutr.* 74(6): 714–722.

Kerr DS 2010. Treatment of mitochondrial electron transport chain disorders: a review of clinical trials over the past decade. *Mol. Genet Metab.* 99(3): 246–55.

Kiefer C, Hessel S, Lampert SM, *et al.* 2001. Identification and characterization of a mammalian enzyme catalyzing the asymmetric oxidative cleavage of provitamin A. *J. Biol. Chem.* 276(17): 14110–14116.

Koushik A, Hunter D, Spiegelman D, *et al.* 2006. Intake of the major carotenoids and the risk of epithelial ovarian cancer in a pooled analysis of 10 cohort studies. *Int. J. Cancer* 119(9): 2148–54.

Kowdley K, Mason J, Meydani S, Cornwall S, and Grand RJ 1992. Vitamin E deficiency and impaired cellular immunity related to intestinal fat malabsorption. *Gastroenterology* 102: 2139–42.

Laguna TA, Sontag MK, Osberg I, *et al.* 2008. Decreased total serum coenzyme-Q_{10} concentrations: a longitudinal study in children with cystic fibrosis. *J. Pediatr.* 153(3): 402–7.

Langlois M, Duprez D, Delanghe J *et al.* 2001. Serum vitamin C concentration is low in peripheral arterial disease and is associated with inflammation and severity of atherosclerosis. *Circulation* 103(14): 1863–1868.

Lee HP, Casadesus G, Zhu X, *et al.* 2009. All-trans retinoic acid as a novel therapeutic strategy for Alzheimer's disease. *Expert Rev Neurother* 9(11): 1615–21.

Lee IM, Cook NR, Gaziano JM, *et al.* 2005. Vitamin E in the primary prevention of cardiovascular disease and cancer: the Women's Health Study: a randomized controlled trial. *JAMA* 294(1): 56–65.

Lonn E, Bosch J, Yusuf S, *et al.* 2005. Effects of long-term vitamin E supplementation on cardiovascular events and cancer: a randomized controlled trial. *JAMA* 293(11): 1338–1347.

Machlin LJ, and Bendich A 1987. Free radical tissue damage: Protective role of antioxidant micronutrients. *FASEB J.* 1: 441–445.

Mahfouz MM, Zhou SQ, and Kummerow FA 2009. Vitamin B6 compounds are capable of reducing the superoxide radical and lipid peroxide levels induced by H_2O_2 in vascular endothelial cells in culture. *Int. J. Vitam. Nutr. Res.* 79(4): 218–29.

McNeil JJ, Robman L, Tikellis G, Sinclair MI, McCarty CA, and Taylor HR 2004. Vitamin E supplementation and cataract: randomized controlled trial. *Ophthalmology.* 111(1): 75–84.

Meydani SN, Leka LS, Fine BC, *et al.* 2004. Vitamin E and respiratory tract infections in elderly nursing home residents: a randomized controlled trial. *JAMA* 292(7): 828–836.

Miller J, and Gallo RL 2010. Vitamin D and innate immunity. *Dermatol Ther.* 23(1): 13–22.

Mohsen S, Mckinney K, and Shanti S 2008. Vitamin A toxicity. Challem, Jack, Caution Urged with Vitamin A in Pregnancy: But Beta-Carotene is Safe, The Nutrition Reporter Newsletter, 1995, retrieved 20 June 2007. http://www.thenutritionreporter.com

Murray M, Michael J, and Pizzorno J 1997. Encyclopedia of Natural Medicine (Revised 2nd Edition) Three Rivers Press. ISBN 0761511571.

Nimptsch K, Rohrmann S, Kaaks R, and Linseisen J 2010. Dietary vitamin K intake in relation to cancer incidence and mortality: results from the Heidelberg cohort of the European Prospective Investigation into Cancer and Nutrition (EPIC-Heidelberg). *Am J Clin Nutr.* 91(5): 1348–58.

Pan Y, and Jackson RT 2009. Dietary phylloquinone intakes and metabolic syndrome in US young adults. *J. Am. Coll. Nutr.* 28(4): 369–79.

Panagiotakos DB, Antonopoulou S, Pitsavos C, and Stefanadis C 2008. Dietary choline and betaine intakes in relation to concentrations of inflammatory markers in healthy adults: the ATTICA study. *Am J Clin Nutr.* 87(2): 424–30.

Paolisso G, D'Amore A, Galzerano D, *et al.* 1993. Daily vitamin E supplements improve metabolic control but not insulin secretion in elderly type II diabetic patients. *Diabetes Care* 16(11): 1433–1437.

Paolisso G, D'Amore A, Giugliano D, *et al.* 1993. Pharmacologic doses of vitamin E improve insulin action in healthy subjects and non-insulin-dependent diabetic patients. *Am. J. Clin. Nutr.* 57(5): 650–656.

Paolisso G, Di Maro G, Galzerano D, *et al.* 1994. Pharmacological doses of vitamin E and insulin action in elderly subjects. *Am J Clin Nutr.* 59(6): 1291–1296.

Patil SM, Chaudhuri D, and Dhanakshirur GB 2009. Role of alpha-tocopherol in cardiopulmonary fitness in endurance athletes, cyclists. *J Physiol Pharmacol.* 53(4): 375–9.

Prasad K 2010. Effect of chronic administration of vitamin E on the hemopoietic system in hypercholesterolemia. *Mol Cell Biochem.* (Epub ahead of print).

Preynat A, Lapierre H, Thivierge MC, *et al.* 2010. Effects of supplementary folic acid and vitamin B(12) on hepatic metabolism of dairy cows according to methionine supply. *J Dairy Sci.* 93(5): 2130–42.

Reaven PD, Herold DA, Barnett J, and Edelman S 1995. Effects of vitamin E on susceptibility of low-density lipoprotein and low-density lipoprotein subfractions to oxidation and on protein glycation in NIDDM. *Diabetes Care.* 18(6): 807–816.

Russel RM, 2002. Beta-carotene and lung cancer. *Pure Appl. Chem.* 74(8): 1461–1467.

Salobir J, Zontar TP, Levart A, and Rezar V 2010. The comparison of black currant juice and vitamin E for the prevention of oxidative stress. *Int. J. Vitam. Nutr. Res.* 80(1): 5–11.

Sánchez-Moreno C, Jiménez-Escrig A, and Martín A 2009. Stroke: roles of B vitamins, homocysteine and antioxidants. *Nutr. Res. Rev*. 22(1): 49–67.

Sasaki T, Yukizane T, Atsuta H, *et al.* 2010. A case of thiamine deficiency with psychotic symptoms-blood concentration of thiamine and response to therapy. *Seishin Shinkeigaku Zasshi*. 112(2): 97–110.

Sauberlich H, 1997. A history of scurvy and vitamin C. *In*: Packer L, and Fuchs J *Eds*. Vitamin C in health and disease. New York: Marcel Decker Inc. pp. 1–24.

Schultink W, 2002. Use of under-five mortality rate as an indicator for vitamin A deficiency in a population. Proceedings of the XX International vitamin A Consultative Group Meeting. *J Nutr*. 132: 2881S–2883S.

Semba RD 1999. Vitamin A as "Anti-Infective" Therapy, 1920–1940. *J. Nutr.* 129: 783–791.

Sen CK, Khanna S, and Roy S 2006. Tocotrienols: vitamin E beyond tocopherols. *Life Sci.* 78: 2088–98.

Slatore CG, Littman AJ, Au DH, Satia JA, and White E 2008. Long-term use of supplemental multivitamins, vitamin C, vitamin E, and folate does not reduce the risk of lung cancer. *Am. J. Respir. Crit. Care Med.* 177(5): 524–530.

Sohal RS, Kamzalov S, Sumien N, *et al.* 2006. Effect of coenzyme Q_{10} intake on endogenous coenzyme Q content, mitochondrial electron transport chain, antioxidative defenses, and life span of mice. *Free Radic. Biol. Med.* 40(3): 480–487.

Sommer A, 2008. Vitamin A deficiency and clinical disease: An historical overview. *J Nutr.* 138: 1835–1839.

Stahl W, Heinrich U, Jungmann H, *et al.* 1998. Increased dermal carotenoid levels assessed by noninvasive reflection spectrophotometry correlate with serum levels in women ingesting beta carotene. *J. Nutr.* 128(5): 903–7.

Stephen R, and Utecht T 2001. Scurvy identified in the emergency department: a case report. *J Emerg Med*. 21(3): 235–237.

Stone Brad. Vitamin A and Birth Defects, 6 October 1995, retrieved 20 June 2007. http://www.fda.gov.bbs.topics

Sudfeld C, Navar A, and Halsey N 2010. Effectiveness of measles vaccination and vitamin A treatment. *Int. J. Epidemiol*. 39(Suppl 1): i48–55.

Tanumihardjo S, 2002. Factors influencing the conversion of carotenoids to retinol: bioavailability to bioconversion to bioefficacy. *Int. J. Vit. Nutr. Res.* 72(1): 40–5.

Tanvetyanon T, and Bepler G 2008. Beta-carotene in multivitamins and the possible risk of lung cancer among smokers versus former smokers: a meta-analysis and evaluation of national brands. *Cancer* 113(1): 150–7.

Tarwadi K, and Agte V 2004. Linkages of antioxidant, micronutrient and socio-economic status with the degree of oxidative stress and lens opacity in Indian cataract patients. *Nutrition*, 20(3): 261–267.

Taylor A, Jacques PF, Chylack LT Jr, *et al.* 2002. Long-term intake of vitamins and carotenoids and odds of early age-related cortical and posterior subcapsular lens opacities. *Am. J. Clin. Nutr.* 75(3): 540–549.

Terwecoren A, Steen E, Benoit D, *et al.* 2009. Ischemic stroke and hyperhomocysteinemia: truth or myth? *Acta Neurol. Belg.* 109(3): 181–8.

Thompson J, and Manore M 2005. Nutrients involved in antioxidant function. Nutrition: An Applied Approach. Pearson Education Inc. Publishers. 8: 276–283.

Traber MG, 2006. Vitamin E. *In*: Bowman BA, and Russell RM *Eds*. Present Knowledge in Nutrition. 9th ed. Vol. 1. Washington, D.C.: ILSI Press. 2: 211–219.

Traber MG 2006. Vitamin E. *In*: Shils ME, Shike M, Ross AC, Caballero B, and Cousins R *Eds*. Modern Nutrition in Health and Disease. 10th ed. Baltimore, MD: Lippincott Williams & Wilkins, pp. 396–411.

Traber MG, 2007. Vitamin E regulatory mechanisms. *Annu. Rev. Nutr.* 27: 347–62.

Ulvik A, Ebbing M, Hustad S, *et al.* 2010. Long- and short-term effects of tobacco smoking on circulating concentrations of B vitamins. *Clin. Chem.* 56(5): 755–63.

Verhagen H, Buijsse B, Jansen E, and Bueno-de-Mesquita B 2006. The state of antioxidant affairs. *Nutr. Today* 41: 244–50.

Vitamin E: Hope or Hopeless, in the Spring/Summer 2000 issue of the Linus Pauling Institute Newsletter.

Wang L, Manson JE, Song Y, and Sesso HD 2010. Systematic review: Vitamin D and calcium supplementation in prevention of cardiovascular events. *Ann Intern. Med.* 152(5): 315–23.

Weinstein M, Babyn P, and Zlotkin S 2001. An orange a day keeps the doctor away: scurvy in the year 2000. *Pediatrics* 108(3): E55.

West AL, Oren GA, and Moroi SE 2006. Evidence for the use of nutritional supplements and herbal medicines in common eye diseases. *Am. J. Ophthalmol* 141(1): 157–166.

Xia W, Zhou Y, Sun C, *et al.* 2010. A preliminary study on nutritional status and intake in Chinese children with autism. *Eur. J. Pediatr*. (Epub ahead of print).

Xu X, Gammon MD, Zeisel SH, *et al.* 2008. Choline metabolism and risk of breast cancer in a population-based study. *The FASEB J* 22(6): 2045–52.

Xu X, Gammon MD, Zeisel SH, *et al.* 2009. High intakes of choline and betaine reduce breast cancer mortality in a population-based study. *FASEB J.* 23(11): 4022–8.

Yamamoto T, Jaroenporn S, Pan L, *et al.* 2009. Effects of pantothenic acid on testicular function in male rats. *J. Vet. Med. Sci.* 71(11): 1427–32.

Ye Z, and Song H 2008. Antioxidant vitamins intake and the risk of coronary heart disease: meta-analysis of cohort studies. *Eur. J. Cardiovasc. Prev. Rehabil.* 15(1): 26–34.

Yvan-Charvet L, Kling J, Pagler T, *et al.* 2010. Cholesterol efflux potential and anti-inflammatory properties of high-density lipoprotein after treatment with Niacin or Anacetrapib. *Arterioscler Thromb Vasc Biol*. (Epub ahead of print)

Zamin I Jr, Mattos AA, Mattos AZ, *et al.* 2010. The vitamin E reduces liver lipoperoxidation and fibrosis in a model of nonalcoholic steatohepatitis. *Arq Gastroenterol*. 47(1): 86–92.

3

Minerals as Important Component of Our Diet

Dietary minerals are the inorganic nutrients, such as calcium, magnesium, potassium, sodium, zinc, and iodine required by human body. The minerals may be already present in the food (*e.g.*, calcium in dairy milk) or added (*e.g.*, orange juice fortified with calcium, salt fortified with iodine, iodized salt). The dietary minerals have importance due to their support to the biochemical reactions of metabolism with the required elemental components. Appropriate intake levels of certain inorganic components are required to maintain optimal health. A healthful, balanced diet can meet all the body's mineral requirements.

Trace elements in the 4 food classes (Tarwadi and Agte, 2007)

Food class	*Zinc mg %*	*Copper mg %*	*Iron mg %*	*Manganese mg%*	*Selenium mg%*
Fruit - Veg.	0.26 ± 0.09	0.05 ± 0.02	1.66 ± 0.68	0.79 ± 0.6	0.07 ± 0.04
Root - Veg.	0.39 ± 0.27	0.02 ± 0.12	1.10 ± 0.97	2.58 ± 0.99	0.17 ± 0.12
Fruits	0.11 ± 0.14	0.02 ± 0.02	0.23 ± 0.27	0.18 ± 0.18	0.05 ± 0.04
GLV	0.09 ± 0.05	0.03 ± 0.02	7.0 ± 7.5	0.43 ± 0.26	0.05 ± 0.01

Plate 8

Humans require about 25 minerals for normal body function and good health, 16 of which are essential nutrients and must be supplied by the diet. There are two groups of minerals. Major minerals (macrominerals, macroelements or bulk minerals) are needed in the diet in amounts of 100 milligrams (mg) or more each day. They include calcium, magnesium, sodium, potassium, phosphorus and chlorine. Acute imbalances of these minerals can be potentially fatal, although nutrition is rarely the cause of these problems. Micronutrients are (also known as trace minerals) iron, cobalt, chromium, copper, iodine, manganese, selenium, zinc, and molybdenum. They are dietary minerals needed by the human body in very small amounts (generally less than 100 mg/day) as opposed to macronutrients which are required in larger quantities (Plate 8).

Important aspects of majority of minerals have been briefly discussed along with detailed discussions on some important trace metals *i.e.* iron, copper, manganese and selenium and a more exhaustive review for zinc.

IRON

Iron is a key element in the metabolism of almost all living organisms. In humans, iron is an essential component of hemoglobin and several other proteins and enzymes (Wood *et al.,* 2006; Beard *et al.,* 1997). Heme is an iron-containing compound found in a number of biomolecules. Hemoglobin and myoglobin are heme-containing proteins for transport and storage of oxygen. Hemoglobin is the chief protein found in red blood cells and represents about two thirds of the body's iron. The vital role of hemoglobin in transporting oxygen from the lungs to the rest of the body is derived from it's unique ability to acquire oxygen in contact with the lungs and release oxygen to the tissues. Myoglobin functions in the transport and short term storage of oxygen in muscle cells, (Yip and Dallman, 1996; Brody, 1999).

Cytochromes are heme containing biomolecules that have important roles in mitochondrial electron transport critical to cellular energy production. Cytochrome P450 is a family of enzymes that function in the metabolism of a number of important biomolecules, as well as the detoxification and metabolism of drugs and pollutants. Nonheme iron-containing enzymes, such as NADH dehydrogenase and succinate dehydrogenase, are also critical to energy metabolism (Yip and Dallman, 1996). Catalase and peroxidases are heme containing enzymes that protect cells against the accumulation of hydrogen peroxide, a highly damaging reactive oxygen species (ROS), by catalyzing a reaction that converts hydrogen peroxide to water and oxygen. As part of the immune response, some white blood cells engulf bacteria and expose them to ROS in order to kill them. The synthesis of one such ROS, hypochlorous acid, by neutrophils is catalyzed by the heme-containing enzyme myeloperoxidase (Yip and Dallman, 1996; Brody, 1999). Ribonucleotide reductase is an iron-dependent enzyme that is required for DNA synthesis (Beard, 1997; Fairbank, 1999).

Vitamin A deficiency may trigger iron deficiency anemia (IDA) and it's supplementation has beneficial effects in IDA by improving iron status of children and pregnant women. The combination of vitamin A and iron has been more effective than either iron or vitamin A individually (Suharno *et al.,* 1993). Adequate copper nutritional status appears to be necessary for normal iron metabolism and red blood cell formation. Anemia is a clinical sign of copper deficiency. Animal studies demonstrate a role for copper in iron absorption (Vulpe *et al.,* 1999), and iron has been found to accumulate in the livers of copper deficient animals, indicating that copper is required for iron transport to the bone marrow for red blood cell formation (Turnland, 2006).

Three levels of iron deficiency are generally identified as in Fig. 1:

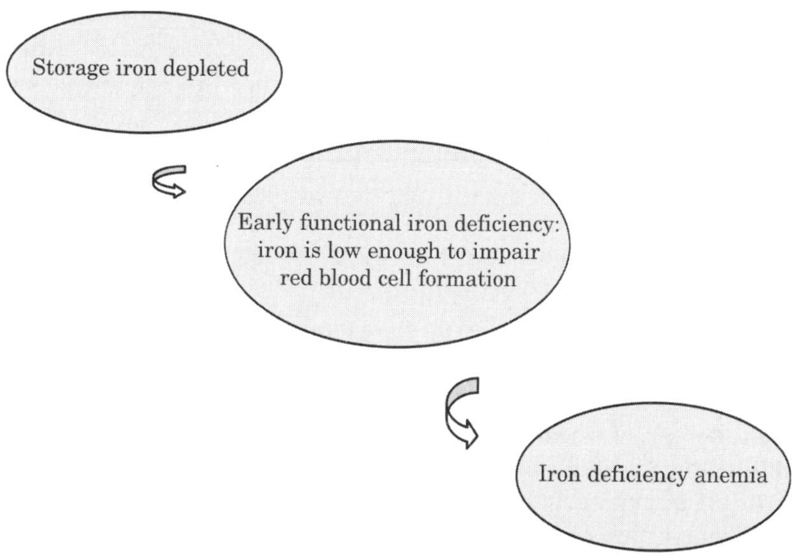

Fig. 1: Iron-deficiency stages

Iron-deficiency anemia

IDA is a result of low levels of iron to support normal red blood cell formation. It is characterized as microcytic and hypochromic RBCs, with their hemoglobin content lowered. Low red cell count, low hematocrit, and low hemoglobin concentrations are all used in the clinical diagnosis of IDA. Most of common symptoms of iron deficiency are fatigue, rapid heart rate, palpitations, and rapid breathing on exertion. Iron deficiency impairs athletic performance and physical work capacity in several ways. Lactic acid production is also elevated in iron deficiency (Beard, 2001). The ability to maintain a normal body temperature on exposure to cold is also impaired in iron-deficient individuals. Severe iron-deficiency anemia may result in brittle and spoon-shaped nails, sores at the corners of the mouth, taste bud atrophy, and a sore tongue. (Plate 9)

Individuals at increased risk of iron deficiency

- Infants and children between the ages of 6 months and 4 years
- Adolescents, pregnant women
- Individuals with chronic blood loss, celiac disease, Helicobacter pylori infection, gastric bypass surgery
- Vegetarians, vegans

Plate 9

Most observational studies have found relationships between iron deficiency anemia in children and poor cognitive development, poor school performance, and behavior problems. However, it is difficult to separate the effects of iron deficiency anemia from other types of deprivation in such studies, and associated factors may contribute to the linkage between iron deficiency and cognitive deficits (Thomas *et al.*, 2009). A recent systematic review of 17 randomized controlled trials concluded that iron supplementation modestly improves scores of mental development in children over seven years of age but has no effect on mental development of children under the age of 27 months (Sachdev *et al.*, 2005). Iron deficiency has been found to increase the intestinal absorption of lead in humans and animals and the risk of lead poisoning in children. Epidemiological studies provide strong evidence of an association between severe anemia in pregnant women and adverse pregnancy outcomes, such as low birth weight, premature birth, and maternal mortality (Yip, 2000).

Iron is required by most infectious vector's, as well as by the infected host in order to manifest an effective immune response. Sufficient iron is critical to several immune functions, including the differentiation and proliferation of T lymphocytes and the generation of reactive oxygen species (ROS) by iron-dependent enzymes, which are used for killing pathogens. During an acute inflammatory response, serum iron levels decrease while levels of ferritin (the iron storage protein) increase, suggesting that sequestering iron from pathogens is an important host response to infection (Beard, 2001 & 2006), (Table 3.1).

Table 3.1: RDA for iron

Group	*Age group*	*RDA (USA) (mg/day)*	*RDA (Indians) mg/day*
Infants	0–12 months	11	
Children	1–3 years	7	12
Children	4–8 years	10	18 (4–6 yrs)
Children	9–13 years	8	26 (7–9 yrs)
Adolescents	14–18 years	11	19–50 (10–18 yrs)
Adults	>19	8	28–30
Pregnancy	all ages	8	38

Source: FNB, USA (2001) and ICMR, 2004

FOOD SOURCES

The amount of iron in food (or supplements) that is bioavailable and used by the body is based on the iron nutritional status of the individual irrespective of the form of iron to be heme or non heme. Anemic or iron deficient individuals absorb a larger percentage of the iron they consume than individuals who are not anemic and have sufficient iron stores (Yip, 1996; Lynch, 1997). Heme iron available in animal foods is more profounly absorbed and its absorption is less affected by other dietary factors due to different mechanism of absorption than nonheme iron. Plant based foods, dairy products, meat, and iron salts added to foods and supplements are all sources of nonheme iron. The absorption of nonheme iron is strongly influenced by enhancers and inhibitors present in the same meal (Yip, 1996; Lynch, 1997; Fairbanks, 1999) are shown in Figs. 2 and 3.

Medications that alleviate stomach acidity, like as antacids, histamine (H_2) receptor antagonists (*e.g.*, cimetidine, ranitidine), and

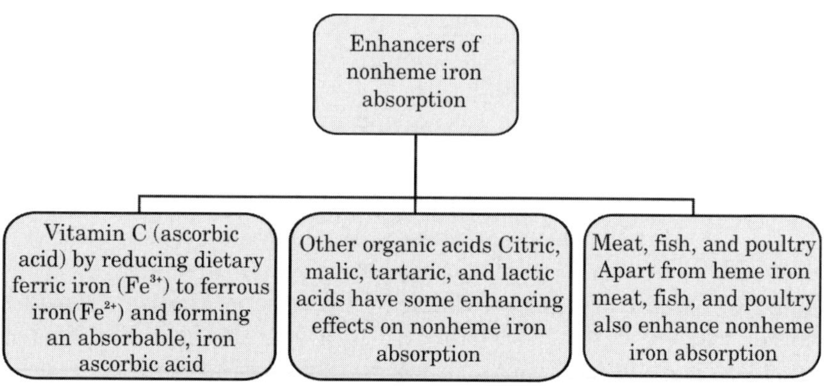

Fig. 2: Enhancers of Iron Absorption

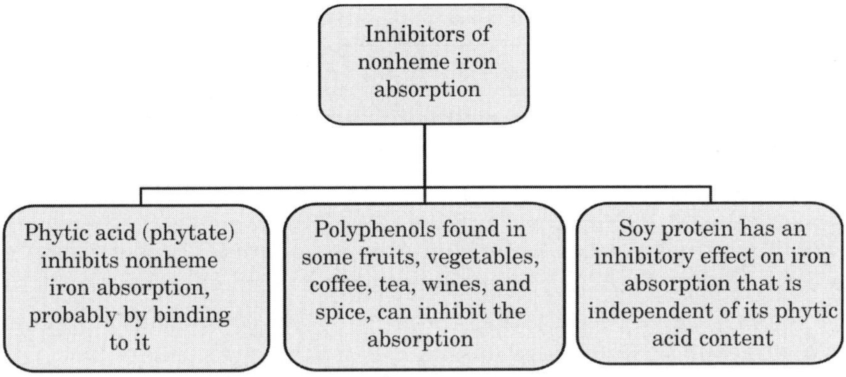

Fig. 3: Inhibitors of Iron Absorption

proton pump inhibitors (*e.g.*, omeprazole, lansoprazole), may impair iron absorption. Iron supplements are indicated for the prevention and treatment of iron deficiency. Individuals who are not at risk of iron deficiency (*e.g.*, adult men and postmenopausal women) should not take iron supplements without an appropriate medication.

IRON OVERLOAD

Several genetic disorders may lead to pathological accumulation of iron in the body. Hereditary hemochromatosis results in iron overload despite of normal iron intake. Iron overload due to prolonged iron supplementation is very rare in healthy individuals without a genetic predisposition. This fact emphasizes the degree to which the body's tight control of intestinal iron absorption protects it from the adverse effects of iron overload (Fairbanks, 1999). However, supplementation of individuals who are not iron deficient should be avoided due to the risk of undetected hereditary hemochromatosis and recent concerns about the more subtle effects of chronic excess iron intake.

Types of Anemia (Nutritional)

Iron Deficiency Anemia

- Iron deficiency causes insufficient hemoglobin production which, in turn, causes anemia and anemia symptoms.

Pernicious Anemia

- It is also known as *megaloblastic*, or vitamin deficiency anemia
- Pernicious anemia is caused by an inability of the intestines to absorb sufficient amounts of vitamin B12 and folic acid which are required in the production of red blood cells.

Plate 10

Iron overload may occur in individuals with acute hereditary anemias that are not caused by iron deficiency. Excessive dietary absorption of iron may occur in response to the body's continued efforts to form red blood cells. Anemic patients at risk of iron overload include those with sideroblastic anemia, pyruvate kinase deficiency, and thalassemia major, especially when they are treated with numerous transfusions. Patients with hereditary spherocytosis and thalassemia minor do not usually develop iron overload unless they are misdiagnosed as having iron deficiency and treated with large doses of iron over many years (Fairbanks 1999). The thalassemias (major and minor) are common in individuals of Mediterranean descent (Pietrangelo, 1998) (Plates 10-11).

Other Types of Anemia

Sickle Cell Anemia

- Sickle cell anemia is characterized by the production of rigid, sickle-shaped red blood cells.
- These abnormal sickle cells break down faster than normal red blood cells, resulting in a chronic shortage of red blood cells and anemia symptoms.

Thalassemia

- *Thalassemia* is one of the genetically inherited types of anemia. Thalassemia occurs when the body's genes, which are responsible for proper hemoglobin production, become damaged or *mutated*. Like sickle cell anemia, thalassemia is one of the hemolytic anemia.

Aplastic Anemia

- Aplastic anemia is one of the rarer types of anemia, occurring when the body makes insufficient red and white blood cells.
- Causes of aplastic anemia include:
  - Radiation therapy, chemotherapy
  - Toxic chemicals, some medications
  - Bone marrow infections.

Plate 11

The oral lethal dose of elemental iron is approximately 200–250 mg/kg of body weight. Symptoms of acute toxicity may occur with iron doses of 20–60 mg/kg of body weight which are nausea, vomiting, abdominal pain, tarry stools, lethargy, weak and rapid pulse, low blood pressure, fever, difficulty breathing, and coma (FNB, 2001).

Epidemiological studies of iron nutritional status and cardiovascular diseases in humans have yielded diverse results. Three large prospective studies found increased dietary heme iron, but not total dietary iron, to be associated with increased risk of myocardial infarction with increased risk of CHD (Ascherio *et al.,* 1994; Klipstein-Grobusch *et al.,* 1999; van der *et al.,* 2005). Although the relationship between iron stores and CHD requires further clarification, it would be safer for those who are not at risk of iron deficiency (*e.g.*, adult men and postmenopausal women) to avoid excess iron intake.

A dramatically increased risk of liver cancer in individuals with cirrhosis due to iron overload in hereditary hemochromatosis has been established. Dietary iron intake appears to be more consistently related to the risk of colorectal cancer than measures of iron status or iron stores and increased red meat consumption has been associated with an increased risk of colorectal cancer (WCRF, 2007). Although this possibility is presently under investigation, the relationship between dietary iron intake, iron stores, and the risk of colorectal cancer remains unclear.

Iron is essential for normal brain and nerve function through its involvement in cellular metabolism, as well as in the synthesis of neurotransmitters and myelin. However, accumulation of excess iron can result in higher oxidative stress, and the brain is particularly susceptible to oxidative damage. Iron accumulation and oxidative injury are presently under consideration as potential contributors to a number of neurodegenerative diseases, such as Alzheimer's disease and Parkinson's disease (Pinero, 2000; Altamura and Muckenthaler, 2009). The abnormal accumulation of iron in the brain does not appear to be a result of higher dietary iron, but rather, a disruption in the complex process of cellular iron regulation. Although the mechanisms for this disruption in iron regulation are not yet known, it is presently an active area of biomedical research (Sayre *et al.,* 2000; Benarroch, 2009) (Plates 12-18).

RECENT REPORTS ON IRON AS MICRONUTRIENT

Evaluation of anemia in children has been reviewed by Janus and Moerschel (2010). As per their opinion, most children with anemia are asymptomatic, and the condition is diagnosed on screening laboratory evaluation. Screening is recommended only for high-risk children. Anemia is classified as microcytic, normocytic, or macrocytic, based on the mean corpuscular volume. Mild microcytic anemia may be treated presumptively with oral iron therapy in children six to 36 months of age who have risk factors for iron deficiency anemia. If the anemia is

Pineapple

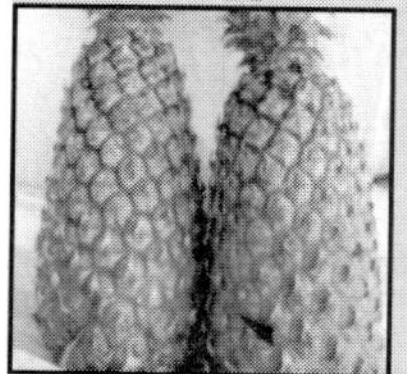

Bajra bhakri

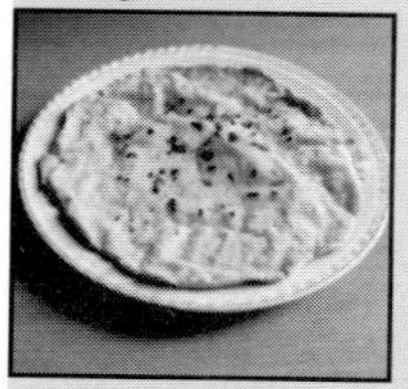

Water melon

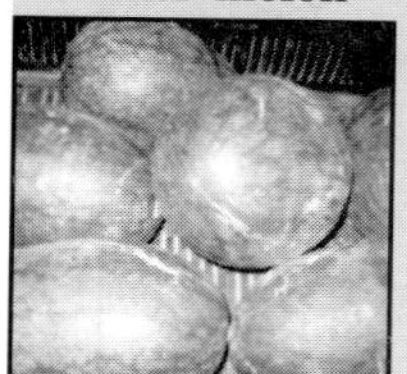

Sources of dietary iron

Food class	*Iron content (mg/100g)*	*Top ranking Indian foods*
Cereals	0.8 – 35	Rice bran, Rice flakes, Bajra
Legumes	1.5 – 10.4	Soybean, Moth beans, Split bengal gram
Other vegetables	0.33 – 7.43	Onion stalks, Green banana, Scarlet beans
Root vegetables	0.2 – 2.6	Mango ginger, Yam, Beetroot
Leafy vegetables	0.8 – 40.0	Amaranth, Cauliflower leaves
Fruits	0.1 – 7.9	Water melon, Peaches, Pineapple
Nuts, oil seeds	0.9 – 100	Garden cress (haliv), Niger seeds (javas), Mustard seeds

Cauliflower leaves

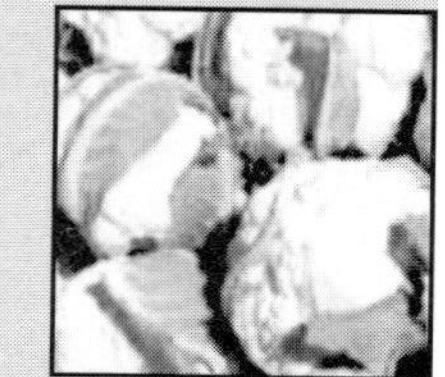

Red amaranthus

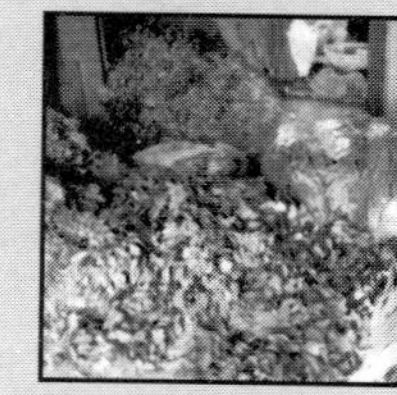

Beet root

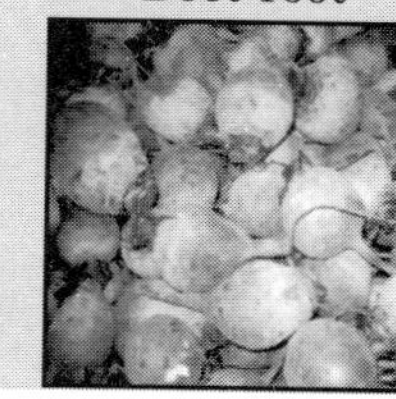

Plate 12

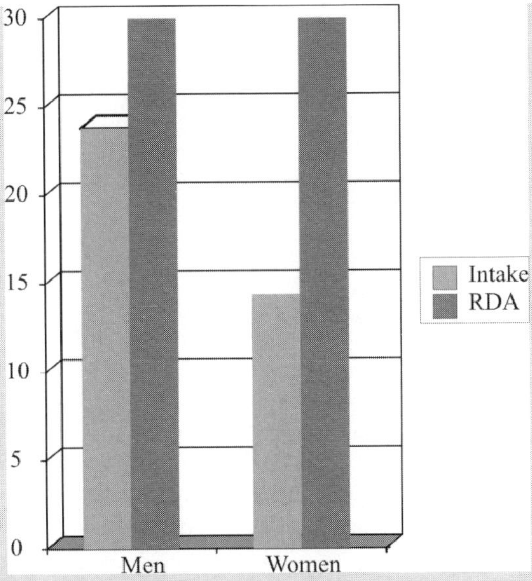

- Intakes of women were 30 to 60 % of the RDA
- When expressed per 1000 k cal, the intakes were 9.5 mg for men & 8 mg for women

Iron intakes (mg/day) of young men & women (Chiplonkar, Agte, Gokhale, 1993)

Plate 13

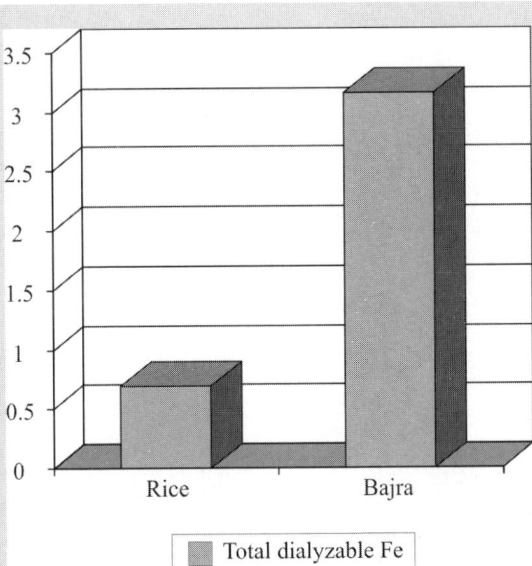

- Total dialyzable iron, was 4.5 times higher in bajra than the rice diets
- Copper and manganese were 2 times higher in bajra diets than the rice diets

Bajra diet

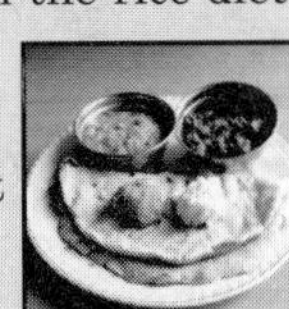

Rice diet

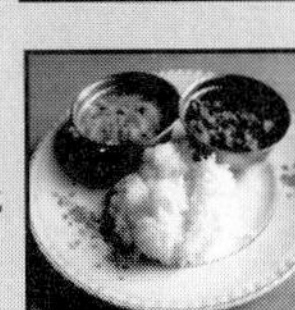

Comparison of rice and bajra diets (Agte *et al.*, 1995)

Plate 14

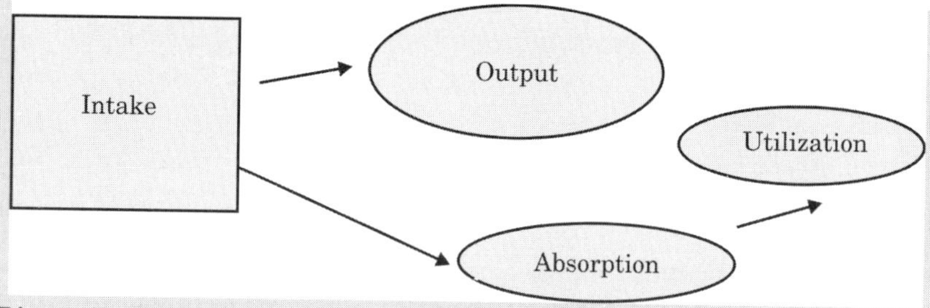

Bioavailability of iron a portion of the total iron content which gets absorbed by human body and utilized

Methods for estimating micronutrient bioavailability

- *In vitro methods*: % Ionisability, % Dialisability
- *Cell models*: Inverted intestinal loops, Caco 2 cell culture in two compartmental system
- *Animal models*: Balance studies, tissue uptakes using rats and mice
- *Human trials*: Balance studies, changes in blood profiles in healthy adults

Plate 15

- ***Enhancers***: vitamin C rich fruits and vegetables

Lemon
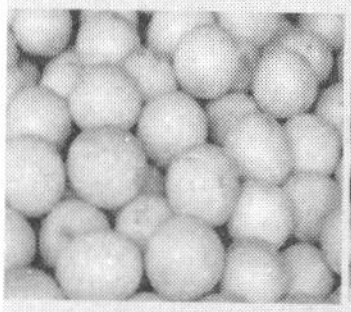
Amla
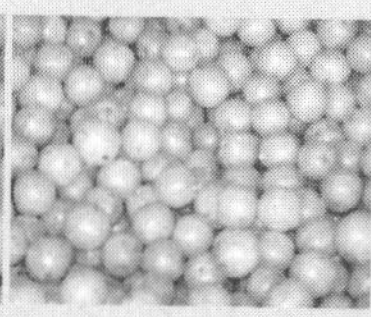
Orange
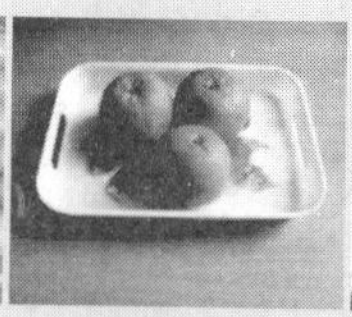
Cauliflower
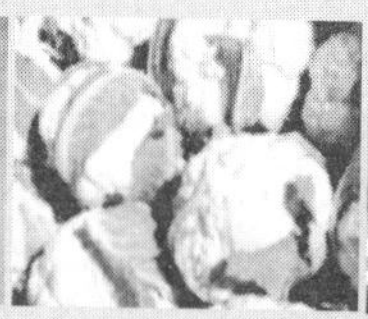
Capsicum
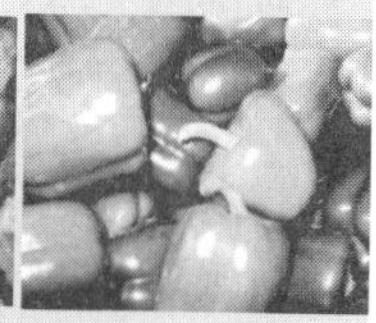

- ***Inhibitors***: foods rich in phytic acid and tannins

Tea
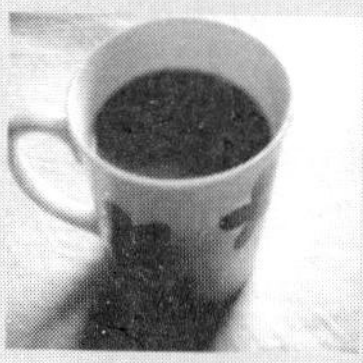
Coffee
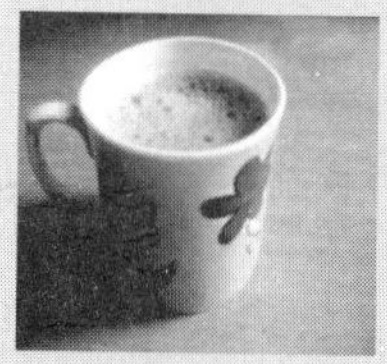
Cereal bran
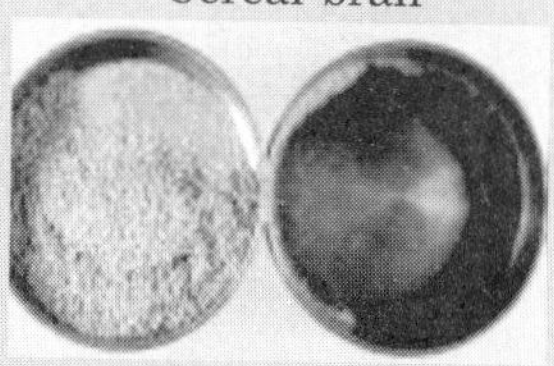

Foods affecting iron bioavailability

Plate 16

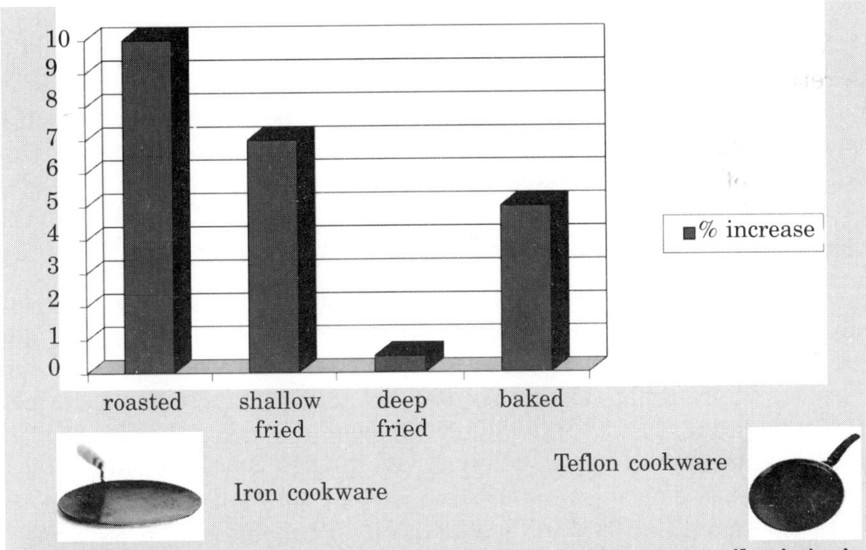

% increase in ionizable iron content due to use of iron utensils vis-à-vis teflon coated nonstickwares (Kakade V and Agte, 1997)

Plate 17

Idli

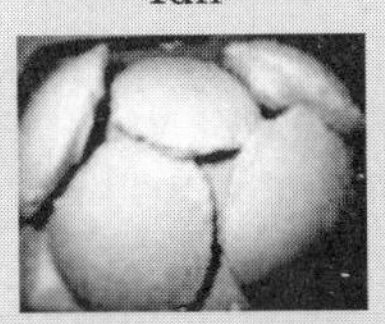

Dosa

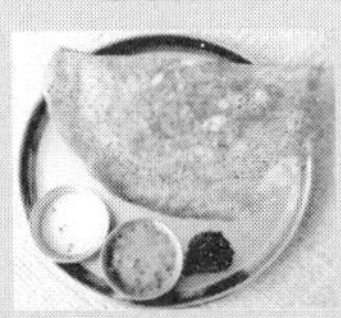

Dhokla

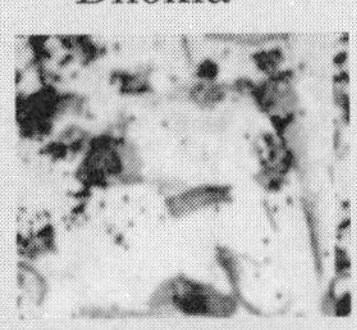

Bread

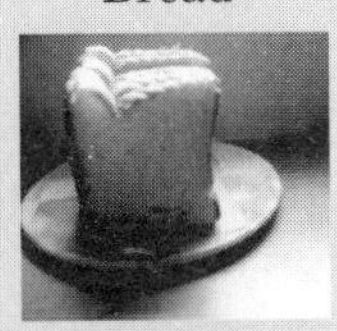

Consumption of naturally fermented (natural flora) foods like idli and dosa, fermented foods using curds (lactic acid bacteria) like dhokla and those using yeast like bread help to increase zinc and iron bioavailability. (Agte *et al.*, 1997)

Keeping the wheat or jowar flour batter for 2 hours prior to roti making increases zinc and iron solubility by 40% (Agte and Joshi, 1992)

Chapati

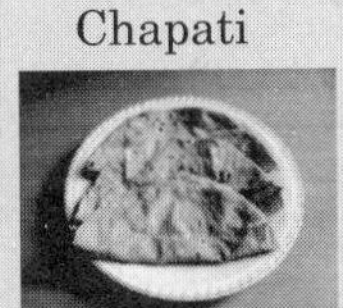

Jowar roti

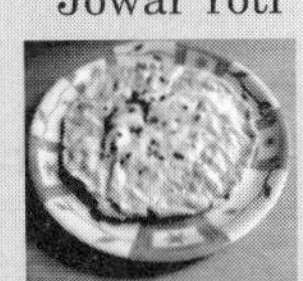

Strategies for improving iron and zinc bioavailability

Plate 18

acute or is unresponsive to iron therapy, the patient should be evaluated for gastrointestinal blood loss. Other tests used in the evaluation of microcytic anemia include serum iron studies, lead levels, and hemoglobin electrophoresis. Normocytic anemia may be caused by chronic disease, hemolysis, or bone marrow disorders. Workup of normocytic anemia is based on bone marrow function as determined by the reticulocyte count. If the reticulocyte count is elevated, the patient should be evaluated for blood loss or hemolysis. A low reticulocyte count suggests aplasia or a bone marrow disorder. Common tests used in the evaluation of macrocytic anemias include vitamin B12 and folate levels, and thyroid function testing. A peripheral smear can provide additional information in patients with anemia of any morphology.

Uncertainty exists regarding the effects of iron supplementation on neurodevelopmental outcomes in the absence of anemia. In one systematic review, MEDLINE, EMBASE, and The Cochrane Library were searched through December 2009 for randomized controlled trials (RCTs). None of 5 RCTs individually showed a beneficial effect of iron supplementation during early life on the Mental Developmental Index of the Bayley Scales of Infant Development at different ages throughout the first 18 months. Meta-analysis of limited available evidence suggests that iron supplementation in infants may positively influence children's psychomotor development, whereas it does not seem to alter their mental development or behavior (Szajewska, 2010).

Metal-mediated oxidation by Fenton chemistry is a common feature for all disorders which take part in a self-amplifying damaging mechanism, leading to neurodegeneration. Neurodegenerative diseases constitute a worldwide health problem. Metals like iron and copper are essential for life, but they are also involved in several neurodegenerative mechanisms such as protein aggregation, free radical generation and oxidative stress. The role of Fe and Cu, their pathogenic mechanisms and possible therapeutic relevance have been examined regarding four of the most common neurodegenerative diseases, Alzheimer's, Parkinson's and Huntington's diseases as well as amyotrophic lateral sclerosis along with the therapeutic strategies tested, mainly using metal chelating drugs. Metal accumulation within the nervous system observed in those diseases could be the result of compensatory mechanisms to improve metal availability for physiological processes (Rivera-Mancía *et al.,* 2010).

Another study has also suggested that iron-induced oxidative stress can play a key role in the pathogenesis of several neurodegenerative diseases. Iron progressively accumulates in the brain both during normal aging and neurodegenerative processes. However, iron accumulation occurs without the concomitant increase in tissue ferritin, which could increase the risk of oxidative stress. Moreover, high iron concentrations in the brain have been consistently observed in Alzheimer's disease (AD) and Parkinson's disease (PD). In this regard, metalloneurobiology has become extremely important in understanding the role of iron in the onset and progression of neurodegenerative diseases. The characterization of the mechanisms involved in high iron induced in neuronal dysfunction and death is central to understanding the pathology of a number of neurodegenerative disorders (Salvador, 2010).

Role of iron metabolism in the retina and in the lens and its relation to their respective age-related pathologies, macular degeneration (AMD) and cataract (ARC) has been reviewed by García-Castiñeiras (2010) paying particular attention to the transport of iron through the blood-retinal barrier and through the lens epithelial cell barrier, to the immunochemistry of iron-related proteins and their expression in both the retina and the lens, and to the nature of the photochemical damage caused by UV light on both tissues. In this review both AMD and ARC are recognized as multifactorial diseases with an important photoxidative component, and exhibiting a remarkable similitude of altered local iron metabolism.

Helicobacter pylori (HP) infection causes morbidity in several systems, especially in the gastrointestinal tract. The prevalence of disease is inversely related to social-economic and developmental status. It is more common in the developing than in developed countries. In the countries where social-economic status is low, not only HP infection,

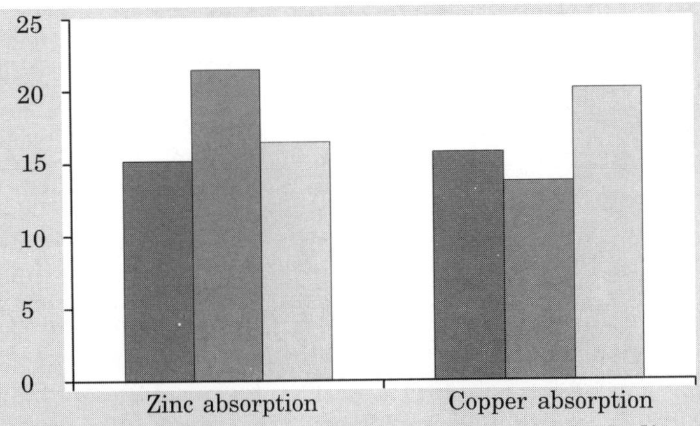

Apparent absorption of Copper and Zinc of young Indian men from composite vegetarian diets was 15 to 20% which is nearly 1/3 that for Western, animal food based, diets (Agte *et al.*, 1994)

Plate 19

but also malnutrition and growth failure have a higher prevalence. Relationship between HP infections and micronutrients, has been reviewed by Akcam (2010). Published studies reveal some evidence that HP has a negative effect on iron, vitamin B12 and vitamin C metabolism, but its influence on others is not clear.

Thus, iron is required for a number of vital functions, including growth, reproduction, healing, and immune function.

COPPER

Copper (Cu) is an essential trace element for humans and animals. The ability of copper to easily accept and donate electrons explains its important role in oxidation-reduction reactions and in scavenging reactive free radicals (Linder and Hazegh-Azam, 1996). Copper is a critical functional component of a number of essential enzymes known as cuproenzymes.

Table 3.2: Copper containing enzymes and their functions

Cuproenzymes	*Function*
Cytochrome c oxidase	A critical role in cellular energy production
Lysyl oxidase,	Required for the cross-linking of collagen and elastin,
Dopamine-b-monooxygenase	catalyzes the conversion of dopamine to the neurotransmitter norepinephrine
Monoamine oxidase (MAO)	Plays a role in the metabolism of the neurotransmitters norepinephrine, epinephrine, and dopamine and in the degradation of the neurotransmitter serotonin
Tyrosinase,	Is required for the formation of the pigment melanin
Superoxide dismutase (SOD)	Functions as an antioxidant by catalyzing the conversion of superoxide radicals (free radicals or ROS) to hydrogen peroxide

Ceruloplasmin may function as an antioxidant in two different ways. Unbound copper and iron ions are powerful catalysts of free radical damage. By binding copper, ceruloplasmin prevents free copper ions from catalyzing oxidative damage. The ferroxidase activity of ceruloplasmin (oxidation of ferrous iron) facilitates iron loading onto its transport protein, transferrin, and may prevent free ferrous ions (Fe^{2+}) from participating in harmful free radical generating reactions (Johnson *et al.*, 1992). Copper-dependent transcription factors regulate transcription of specific genes. Thus, cellular copper levels may affect the synthesis of proteins by enhancing or inhibiting the transcription of specific genes. Genes regulated by copper-dependent transcription factors include genes for copper/zinc superoxide dismutase (Cu/Zn SOD), catalase (another antioxidant enzyme), and proteins related to the cellular storage of copper (Uauy *et al.,* 1998).

Clinically evaluated or frank copper deficiency is relatively uncommon. Serum copper levels and ceruloplasmin levels may fall to 30% of normal in cases of severe copper deficiency. One of the most common clinical symptom of copper deficiency is an anemia that is unresponsive to iron therapy but corrected by copper supplementation. Copper deficiency may also result in abnormally low numbers of white blood cells known as neutrophils (neutropenia), a condition that may be accompanied by increased susceptibility to infection. Osteoporosis and other abnormalities of bone development related to copper deficiency are most common in copper-deficient low-birth weight infants and young children. Uncommon features of copper deficiency are loss of pigmentation, neurological symptoms, and impaired growth (Turnlund *et al.,* 2006; Uauy *et al.,* 1998). Cow's milk is relatively low in copper, and cases of copper deficiency have been reported in high-risk infants and children fed only cow's milk (Plate 19).

High-risk individuals of copper deficiency

Premature infants (especially those with low-birth weight); Infants with prolonged diarrhea; Infants and children recovering from malnutrition; Individuals with malabsorption syndromes; including celiac disease, sprue, and short bowel syndrome; Individuals receiving intravenous total parenteral nutrition or other restricted diets; Cystic fibrosis patients may also be at increased risk of copper insufficiency (Percival *et al.*, 1999).

The Recommended Dietary Allowance (RDA)

Copper is abundant in a wide variety of foods and is most plentiful in organ meats, shellfish, nuts, and seeds. Wheat bran cereals and whole grain products are also good sources of copper. Some foods that are relatively poor in copper are refined cereal flours and their products.

A variety of parameters were used to establish the recommended dietary allowance (RDA) for copper, including plasma copper concentration, serum ceruloplasmin activity, superoxide dismutase activity in red blood cells, and platelet copper concentration (Food and Nutrition Board, 2001). The RDA for copper reflects the results of depletion-repletion studies and is based on the prevention of deficiency (Table 3.3).

Table 3.3: RDA for Copper

Group	*Age group*	*RDA (mcg/day)*
Infants	0–12 months	200 (AI)
Children	1–3 years	340
Children	4–8 years	440
Children	9–13 years	700
Adolescents	14–18 years	890
Adults	>19	900
Pregnancy	all ages	1,000
Breastfeeding	all ages	1,300

Source: FNB, 2001

Role of copper in disease prevention

In vitro, free copper is known to be a pro-oxidant and is frequently used to produce oxidation of low density lipoprotein (LDL) and there is little evidence that copper or ceruloplasmin promotes LDL oxidation in the human body. Additionally, the cuproenzymes, superoxide dismutase and ceruloplasmin, are known to have antioxidant properties, leading some researchers to propose that copper deficiency rather than excess copper increases the risk of cardiovascular diseases (Jones *et al.*, 1997). However, some epidemiological studies have found higher serum copper levels to be associated with higher risk of cardiovascular disease.

A prospective study in the U.S. evaluated serum copper levels in more than 4,500 men and women 30 years of age and older (Ford, 2000) when after adjusting for other risk factors of heart disease, those with serum copper levels in the two highest quartiles had a significantly higher risk of dying from CHD. In 60 patients with chronic heart failure serum copper was a predictor of short-term outcome (Malek *et al.*, 2006).

A recent study reported that high serum copper levels were significantly related to a 50% increase in all-cause mortality; however, serum copper was not significantly associated with cardiovascular mortality in this study (Leone *et al.*, 2006). In most of the studies serum copper levels were based on serum ceruloplasmin which is not a sensitive indicator of copper nutritional status since serum ceruloplasmin is

Table 3.4: Some recent studies on copper

Findings	***Reference(s)***
The hypothesis that copper toxicity is the major cause of the epidemic of mild cognitive impairment and Alzheimer's disease in aging population is getting experimental support that the epidemic is associated with the use of copper plumbing, and the taking of copper in multi-mineral supplements	Brewer, 2009
A portion of the superoxide generated at complex III is also released into the mitochondrial intermembrane space, which contains a recently identified copper, zinc superoxide dismutase (Cu,ZnSOD). Deletion of Cu,ZnSOD has been shown to lead to a phenotype of accelerated age-related loss of skeletal muscle mass and function	Jackson, 2009
Although regulators are more concerned with the potential human toxicity arising from excessive Cu intake, the preponderance of evidence suggests that deficiency is more of a public health concern than excess	Stern, 2010
The transition metal copper is an essential trace element involved in many enzymatic processes that require redox-chemistry. The redox-activity of copper is potentially harmful. Severe imbalance of copper homeostasis can occur with some hereditary disorders of copper metabolism.	van den Berghe & Klomp, 2009
Redox properties bestow Cu with capabilities that are simultaneously essential and potentially damaging to the cell. The descriptions of the structural and functional organization of the metallothioneins, Cu is stored by metallothioneins and distributed by specialized chaperones to specific cell targets that make use of its redox properties. Transfer of Cu to newly synthesized cuproenzymes and Cu disposal is performed by the individual or concerted actions of the P-type ATPases ATP7A and ATP7B expressed in tissues. In mammalians, liver is the major captor, distributor and excreter of Cu. Mutations in the P-type ATPases that interfere with their functioning and traffic are cause of the life-threatening Wilson (ATP7B) and Menkes (ATP7A) diseases.	Lalioti *et al.*, 2009

known to increase by 50% or more under trauma, inflammation, or disease. Nevertheless, serum copper was also found to be elevated in patients with rheumatic heart disease (Kosar *et al.,* 2005). In contrast to the epidemiological findings linking serum copper to heart disease, two autopsy studies found copper levels in heart muscle were actually decreased in patients who died of CHD than those who died of other causes (Klevay, 2000). Thus, due to a lack of a reliable biomarker of copper nutritional status, it is unclear whether copper is related to cardiovascular disease.

Copper also plays an important role in the development and functioning of immune system, but the exact mechanism of its action is not yet known. The copper-dependent enzyme, lysyl oxidase, is required for the maturation (cross-linking) of collagen, a key element in the organic matrix of bone.

Copper toxicity is rare in the free-living population. Acute copper poisoning has occurred through the contamination of beverages by storage in copper-containers as well as from contaminated water supplies (Bremner, 1998). Symptoms of acute copper toxicity include abdominal pain, nausea, vomiting, and diarrhea, which help prevent additional ingestion and absorption of copper. More serious signs of acute copper toxicity include severe liver damage, kidney failure, coma, and death. In generally healthy individuals, doses of up to 10 mg/ day have not resulted in liver damage. But, individuals with genetic disorders affecting copper metabolism such as Wilson's disease, Indian childhood cirrhosis, and idiopathic copper toxicosis may be at risk for adverse effects of chronic copper toxicity at significantly lower intake levels. Table 3.4 gives some recent studies on copper.

MANGANESE

Manganese is both nutritionally essential and potentially toxic trace metal since it shows diverse effects of deficiency and toxicity in living organisms. Manganese (Mn) plays an important role in a number of physiological processes either as a constituent or an activator of enzymes such as superoxide dismutase (MnSOD), the principal antioxidant enzyme in the mitochondria which catalyzes the conversion of superoxide radicals to hydrogen peroxide, which can be reduced to water by other antioxidant enzymes.

A number of manganese dependent enzymes play important roles in the metabolism of carbohydrates, amino acids, and cholesterol. Pyruvate carboxylase, and phosphoenolpyruvate carboxykinase (PEPCK), are critical in the production of glucose from non-carbohydrate precursors. Arginase, is required by the liver for the urea cycle, a process that detoxifies ammonia generated during amino acid metabolism. In the brain, glutamine synthetase, converts the amino acid glutamate to glutamine. Glutamate is an excitotoxic neurotransmitter and a precursor to an inhibitory neurotransmitter, gamma-aminobutyric acid (GABA).

Manganese deficiency results in abnormal skeletal development in a number of animal species. Manganese is the preferred cofactor of enzymes called glycosyl transferases required for the synthesis of proteoglycans for the formation of healthy cartilage and bone. Wound healing is a complex process that requires higher production of collagen. Manganese is required for the activation of prolidase, an enzyme that functions to provide the amino acid, proline, for collagen formation in human skin cells. A genetic disorder known as prolidase deficiency results in abnormal wound healing among other problems, and is characterized by abnormal manganese metabolism. Low dietary manganese or low levels of manganese in blood or tissue have been linked with several chronic diseases like osteoporosis, diabetes mellitus, epilepsy.

Estimated normal dietary manganese intakes in the U.S., range from 2.1–2.3 mg/day for men and 1.6–1.8 mg/day for women. People eating vegetarian diets and Western-type diets may have manganese intakes as high as 10.9 mg/day (FNB, 2001). Indian RDA for Mn is 5 mg. Rich sources of manganese include whole grains, nuts, leafy vegetables, and teas. Foods high in phytic acid, such as beans, seeds, nuts, whole grains, and soy products, or foods high in oxalic acid, such as cabbage, spinach, and sweet potatoes, may slightly inhibit manganese absorption. Although teas are rich sources of manganese, the tannins present in tea may moderately reduce the absorption of manganese (Kies, 1994). Intake of other minerals, including iron, calcium, and phosphorus, have been found to lower retention of manganese (FNB, 2001).

Manganese toxicity may result in multiple neurological problems and is a well-recognized health hazard for people who inhale manganese dust, such as welders and smelters (Keen, 1999; FNB, 2001). Unlike ingested manganese, inhaled manganese is transported directly to the brain before it can be metabolized in the liver (Davis, 1998). In its worst form, manganese toxicity can result in a permanent neurological disorder with symptoms similar to those of Parkinson's disease, including tremors, difficulty in walking, and facial muscle spasms. Additionally, environmental or occupational inhalation of manganese can cause an inflammatory response in the lungs (Han *et al.,* 2008). Clinical signs of effects to the lung include cough, acute bronchitis, and decreased lung function (Roels *et al.,* 1987). MMT is a manganese-containing compound used in gasoline as an anti-knock additive. The impact of long-term exposure to low levels of MMT combustion products, however, has not been thoroughly evaluated and will require additional study (Aschner, 2000). Limited evidence suggests that high manganese intakes from drinking water may be associated with neurological symptoms similar to those of Parkinson's disease. U.S., the EPA recommends 0.05 mg/litre as the maximum allowable manganese concentration in drinking water (EPA, 2008).

Manganese neurotoxicity has been documented in individuals receiving total parenteral nutrition, both as a result of excessive manganese in the solution and as an incidental contaminant (Dobson *et al.,* 2004). Neonates are especially prone to manganese-related neurotoxicity (Erickson *et al.,* 2007). Infants receiving manganese-containing TPN can be exposed to manganese concentrations about 100-fold higher than breast-fed infants (Aschner, 2005). Because of potential toxicities, some debate against including manganese in parenteral nutrition (Hardy *et al.,* 2008).

Individuals with increased susceptibility to manganese toxicity

***Chronic liver disease*:** Manganese accumulation in individuals with cirrhosis or liver failure may contribute to neurological problems and Parkinson's disease-like symptoms (Keen, 1999; Hendler and Rorvik, 2001).

***Newborns*:** Due to a increased expression of receptors for the manganese transport protein in developing nerve cells and the immaturity of the liver's bile elimination.

***Children*:** They are more susceptible to any negative, neurotoxic effects of manganese as seen in reported deleterious cognitive and behavioral effects following excessive manganese exposure (Wasserman *et al.,* 2006; Bouchard *et al.,* 2007; Wright *et al.,* 2006).

***Iron-deficient populations*:** Iron deficiency has been shown to increase the risk of manganese accumulation in the brain (Aschner and Dorman, 2006).

Magnesium-containing antacids and laxatives and the antibiotic medication, tetracycline, may decrease the absorption of manganese if taken together with manganese-containing foods or supplements (Hendler and Rorvik, 2001).

Table 3.6: Some recent reports on Manganese

	Findings	*Reference(s)*
Mn status	Determining plasma level of copper, manganese and selenium may contribute to assessing the health and nutritional status of populations. A cross-sectional survey in southern Spain with random blood samples of 340 subjects and food consumption was assessed by 48-h recall, when 9.7% presented hypomanganesemia. Moreover, plasma Mn was directly correlated with the consumption of dairy products.	Sánchez *et al.*, 2010
Mn content	The manganese concentration in different food categories in Meghalaya varied from 2.76–12.50 mg kg(-1) in cereals, 1.8-4.20 mg kg(-1) in leafy vegetables, 0.30–13.50 mg kg(-1) in non leafy vegetables, 0.50-15.30 mg kg(-1) in roots and tubers, 0.70-1.50 mg kg(-1) in fruits and 0.12-0.96 mg kg(-1) in flesh food. The mean dietary intake of Mn was found to be 3.83+/-0.25 mg d(-1) compared to Recommended Dietary Allowances (RDAs) of 2–5 mg d(-1). The daily intake of Manganese by the local tribe population is comparable with the value (3.7 mg d(-1)) recommended by International Commission on Radiological Protection (ICRP) for reference man and lower than the intake value observed for Indian and other Asian population.	Gothankar *et al.*, 2009
	The concentrations of arsenic (As), cadmium (Cd), chromium (Cr), copper (Cu), mercury (Hg), manganese (Mn), nickel (Ni), and lead (Pb) were determined in samples of various edible vegetables (artichoke, cauliflower, lettuce, tomato), fruits (apple, mandarin, orange, pear) and rice grown in soils irrigated with water from the Ebro River in Tarragona Province (Catalonia, Spain).	Ferré-Huguet *et al.*, 2008
Linkages with disease	The association of antioxidants with risk of non-Hodgkin's lymphoma (NHL) overall and for diffuse large B-cell lymphoma (DLBCL) and follicular lymphoma specifically in a prospective cohort of 35,159 Iowa women aged 55-69 years when enrolled at baseline in 1986 was evaluated. The strongest associations of antioxidants with risk of NHL (RR for highest versus lowest quartile; p for trend) were observed for dietary vitamin C (RR=0.78; p=0.044), alpha-carotene (RR=0.71; p=0.015), proanthocyanidins (RR=0.70; p=0.0024) and dietary manganese (RR=0.62; p=0.010).	Thompson *et al.*, 2010
	The association of antioxidant vitamins and trace elements from foods and supplements with risk of rheumatoid arthritis was evaluated in a prospective cohort study of 29,368 women who were aged 55-69 years at baseline in 1986. Through 1997, 152 cases of rheumatoid arthritis were identified. Greater use of supplemental zinc (RR=0.39, 95% CI: 0.17, 0.88; p-trend = 0.03) was inversely associated with rheumatoid arthritis, while any use of supplemental copper (RR=0.54, 95% CI: 0.28, 1.03) and manganese (RR=0.50, 95% CI: 0.23, 1.07) showed suggestive inverse associations with rheumatoid arthritis.	Cerhan *et al.*, 2003

RDA

The adequate intake (AI) for manganese (2.3 mg/day for adult men and 1.8 mg/day for adult women) appears sufficient to prevent deficiency in most individuals. The daily intake of manganese most likely to promote optimum health is unknown. Because of the potential for toxicity and the lack of information regarding benefit, manganese supplementation beyond 2 mg/day is not recommended. There is presently no evidence that the consumption of a manganese-rich plant-based diet results in manganese toxicity. The requirement for manganese is not known to be higher for older adults. However, liver disease is more common in older adults and may increase the risk of manganese toxicity by decreasing the elimination of manganese from the body. Table 3.6 shows some recent reports on Manganese.

SELENIUM

Selenium is a trace mineral essential in small amounts, but which shows toxic effects at high levels. Humans and animals require selenium for the function of a number of selenium-dependent enzymatic proteins known as *selenoproteins*. Although 25 selenoproteins have been identified, the metabolic functions have been identified for only about one-half of them (Gladyshev, 2006). When selenium is present in the soil, plants incorporate it non-specifically into compounds that usually contain sulfur (Rayman, 2000). Selenium is an essential element for normal development, growth, and metabolism because of its role in the regulation of thyroid hormones (Gladyshev, 2006; Bianco and Larsen, 2006) (Table 3.7).

Causes of selenium deficiency

Insufficient selenium intake results in decreased activity of the selenoproteins.

Total parenteral nutrition (TPN) without added selenium for prolonged periods of time. Symptoms include muscular weakness, muscle wasting, and cardiomyopathy (inflammation and damage to the heart muscle).

Keshan disease, a cardiomyopathy affects young women and children in a selenium-deficient region of China (Burk *et al.*, 1999, Foster and Sumar, 1997)

Table 3.7: Role of important selenoproteins

Selenoprotein	***Function***
Antioxidant enzymes: cellular or classical GPx, plasma or extracellular GPx, phospholipid hydroperoxide GPx, gastrointestinal GPx, and olfactory GPx. Sperm mitochondrial capsule selenoprotein, phospholipid hydroperoxide GPx	Glutathione peroxidases(GPx) reduce potentially damaging reactive oxygen species (ROS), such as hydrogen peroxide and lipid hydroperoxides, to harmless products like water and alcohols by coupling their reduction with the oxidation of glutathione
Thioredoxin reductase	Participates in the regeneration of several antioxidants, possibly including vitamin C. Maintenance of thioredoxin in a reduced form by thioredoxin reductase is important for regulating cell growth and viability
Iodothyronine deiodinases (types I, II, and III)	Can both activate and inactivate thyroid hormone by acting on T_3, T_4, or other thyroid hormone metabolites
Selenoprotein P	Found in plasma and also associated with vascular endothelial cells and acts as transport protein for selenium and also functions as an antioxidant that protects endothelial cells from damage induced by such compounds as peroxynitrite, a reactive nitrogen species (RNS) (Burk *et al.*, 2006, Arteel *et al.*, 1999)

Disease preventive role of Selenium

***Immune response*:** Selenium supplementation in individuals who are not diognosed selenium deficient appears to stimulate the immune response (Roy *et al.,* 1994; Kiremidjian-Schumacher *et al.,* 1994; Kiremidjian-Schumacher *et al.,* 2000). Selenium plays a role in regulating the expression of cell-signaling molecules called cytokines, which orchestrate the immune response (Baum *et al.,* 2000).

***Viral infections*:** Selenium deficiency appears to enhance the virulence or progression of some viral infections such as Coxsackievirus (Beck, 2006). As an integral component of glutathione peroxidase and thioredoxin reductase, selenium plays an important role in decreasing oxidative stress in HIV-infected cells and possibly suppressing the rate of HIV replication (Baum and Campa, 2006). Recent research indicates that HIV may be capable of incorporating host selenium into viral selenoproteins that have glutathione-peroxidase activity. Though the significance of these findings requires further clarification, they suggest that both the human immune system and the activity of the virus are affected by selenium nutritional status (Baum and Campa, 2006; Zao *et al.,* 2000; Zang *et al.,* 1999). Selenium supplementation in HIV-infected individuals has been published with controversial results (Constans *et al.,* 1999; Delmas-Beauvieux *et al.,* 1996; Constans *et al.,* 1996; Burbano *et al.,* 2002; Hurwitz *et al.,* 2007).

***Hepatitis infection and cigarette smoking*:** Low dietary selenium intake may heighten cancer risk and increase risk of chronic infection with viral hepatitis B or C which in turn can significantly increase risk of liver cancer (Yu *et al.,* 1999).

***Cancer*:** Selenium supplementation at high levels reduces the incidence of cancer in animals (Combs and Grey, 1998). The evidence indicates that the methylated forms of selenium are the active species against tumors, and these are produced at the greatest amounts with excess selenium intakes (Ip, 1998). The relationships of selenium intake to cancer in humans and selenium status to tumor incidence in animals have been reviewed (Whanger, 2004). Geographic studies have consistently observed higher cancer mortality rates in populations living in areas with low soil selenium and relatively low dietary selenium intakes which are more so for men (Garland *et al.,* 1995). Lower serum selenium levels were associated with an increased risk of lung cancer, and the association was more pronounced in smokers (Knekt *et al.,* 1998). However, a nonsignificant decrease (20% reduction) in lung cancer risk was found when studies assessing selenium status by serum levels were collectively analyzed (Zuo *et al.,* 2004).

Some studies have reported that low dietary selenium intakes are associated with increased risk of prostate cancer (Yoshizawa *et al.,* 1998; Nomura *et al.,* 2000; Brooks *et al.,* 2001). A meta-analysis of 20 epidemiological studies, mainly case-control studies, found that selenium levels in the serum or toenails were significantly lower in those with prostate cancer (Brinkman *et al.,* 2006). However, a recent prospective study in a cohort of over 295,000 men reported that frequent multivitamin use greater than 7 times/week and use of selenium supplements, together, was associated with significant increases in advanced and fatal prostate cancer (Lawson *et al.,* 2007). In the U.S., a double-blind, placebo-controlled study of more than 1,300 older adults with a history of nonmelanoma skin cancer found that supplementation with 200 mcg/day of selenium-enriched yeast for an average of 7.4 years was associated with a 49% decrease in prostate cancer incidence in men (Duffield-Lillico *et al.,* 2003).

***Cardiovascular disease*:** Prospective studies in humans have not demonstrated strong support for the cardioprotective effects of selenium (Salonen *et al.,* 1982; Virtamo *et al.,* 1985; Suadicani *et al.,* 1992; Salvini *et al.,* 1995). In a multi-center study in Europe, toenail selenium levels and risk of myocardial infarction (heart attack) were only associated in the center where selenium levels were the lowest (Kardinaal *et al.,* 1997). While some epidemiological evidence suggests that low levels of selenium (lower than those commonly found in the U.S.) may increase the risk of cardiovascular diseases, definitive evidence regarding the role of selenium in preventing cardiovascular diseases will require controlled clinical trials.

***Type 2 Diabetes Mellitus*:** Lower toenail selenium levels in men were found with type 2 diabetes than in non-diabetic men (Rajpathak *et al.,* 2005); while, higher serum selenium levels in type 2 diabetics are reported (Bleys *et al.,* 2007). Selenium supplementation (200 mcg/day; mean follow-up of 7.7 years) was linked to an increase in prevalence of type 2 diabetes (Stranges *et al.,* 2007). In the Selenium and Vitamin E Cancer Prevention Trial (SELECT), selenium supplementation (200 mcg/day; median follow-up of 5.5 years) was associated with a statistically nonsignificant increased risk of type 2 diabetes (Lippman *et al.,* 2009).

Toxicity

Although selenium is required for health, high doses of selenium can be toxic. The most frequently reported symptoms of selenosis are hair and nail brittleness and loss, gastrointestinal disturbances, skin rashes, a garlic breath odor, fatigue, irritability, and nervous system abnormalities. The Food and Nutrition Board (FNB) of the Institute of Medicine recently set the tolerable upper intake level (UL) for selenium at 400 mcg/day in adults based on the prevention of hair and nail brittleness.

ZINC

Zinc is an essential trace element for animals, plants as well as microorganisms. Clinical zinc deficiency in humans was first described in 1961, when the consumption of diets with low zinc bioavailability due to high phytic acid content was associated with a kind of dwarfism in the Middle East (Prasad *et al.,* 1961). Zinc as a micronutrient for humans catalyzes metabolic reactions through more than 100 enzymes, facilitates protein folding, and helps regulate gene expression including metalloenzymes and metalloenzyme complexes, which are necessary in the metabolism of carbohydrates, fatty acids, proteins and nucleic acids. It is an important factor in the metabolism of neurotransmitters, prostaglandins, and for maintaining brain structure and function. Deficiency of zinc is prevalent worldwide in developing countries affecting nearly 2 billion subjects.

The major observations of zinc deficiency in humans include growth retardation, hypogonadism in males, cell-mediated immune dysfunctions, and cognitive impairment. Zinc not only improves cell mediated immune functions but also acts as an antioxidant and anti-inflammatory agent. Zinc plays multiple roles, especially in pregnant women and children. Although the issue of micronutrient malnutrition has been raised in developing countries, it has been remarked to be prevalent also in developed ones, due to unbalanced nutrition and diets. The important aspects related to zinc micronutrient are: metabolic pathway, daily dosage, health benefits as prophylaxis and therapy of respiratory and digestive ailments in children (Florescu *et al.,* 2009).

Zinc supplementation has proven to be beneficial in the treatment of acute pediatric diarrhea and appears to enhance linear growth. Zinc is essential for normal brain development. Gestational severe zinc deficiency can lead to overt fetal brain malformations. Although not teratogenic, suboptimal zinc nutrition during gestation can have long-term effects on the offspring's nervous system. Zinc deficiency during gestation, even at the marginal levels observed in human populations, could increase the risk for behavioral/neurological disorders in infancy, adolescence, and adulthood (Plate 20, Table 3.8 and Table 3.9).

Numerous aspects of cellular metabolism are zinc-dependent. Zinc plays important roles in growth and development, the immune response, neurological function, and reproduction. On the cellular level, the function of zinc can be divided into three categories: 1) catalytic, 2) structural, and 3) regulatory (Cousins, 2006). Nearly 100 different enzymes depend on zinc for their ability to catalyze vital chemical reactions. Zinc-dependent enzymes can be found in all known classes of enzymes. Zinc plays an important role in the structure of proteins and cell membranes. A finger-like structure, known as a zinc finger motif, stabilizes the structure of a number of proteins. For example, copper provides the catalytic activity for the antioxidant enzyme copper-zinc superoxide dismutase (CuZnSOD), while zinc plays a critical structural role (FNB, 2001; King *et al.*, 2006). The structure and function of cell membranes are also affected by zinc. Loss of zinc from biological membranes increases their susceptibility to oxidative damage and impairs their function (O'Dell 2000). Zinc finger proteins have been found to regulate gene expression by acting as transcription factors (binding to DNA and influencing the transcription of specific genes). Zinc also plays a role in cell signaling and has been found to influence hormone release and nerve impulse transmission. Recently, zinc has been found to play a role in apoptosis (gene-directed cell death), a critical cellular

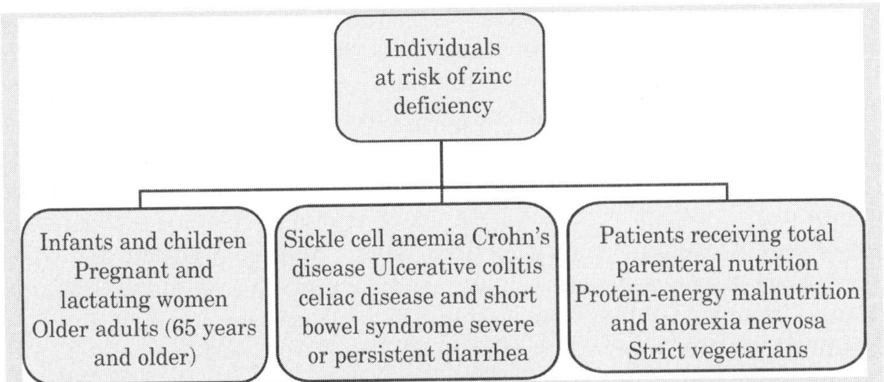

Risk of zinc deficiency

Plate 20

Table 3.8: Stages of zinc deficiency

	Severe zinc deficiency	*Mild zinc deficiency*
Causes	*Genetic*: acrodermatitis enteropathica *Others*: severe burns or prolonged diarrhea	Dietary inadequacy
Symptoms	Slowing or cessation of growth and development delayed sexual maturation characteristic skin rashes, chronic and severe diarrhea, immune system deficiencies, impaired wound healing, diminished appetite, impaired taste sensation, night blindness, swelling and clouding of the corneas, and behavioral disturbances	Impaired physical and neuropsychological development and increased susceptibility to life-threatening infections in young children

regulatory process with implications for growth and development, as well as a number of chronic diseases (Truong-Tran, 2000).

Table 3.9: The Recommended Dietary Allowance (RDA) for Zinc (mg/day)

	Age	*USA (FNB, 2001)*	*India*
Infants	0–1 years	2–3	NA
Children	1–3 years	3–8	NA
Adolescents	14–18 years	9–11	NA
Adults	19 years and older	8–11	15.5

During pregnancy and lactation: +2 mg/day

ZINC DURING GROWTH AND DEVELOPMENT

Significant delays in linear growth and weight gain also, known as growth retardation or failure to thrive, are common in mild zinc deficiency in children. Since the classical studies of zinc deficiency by Prasad (1961), a number of prospective studies of zinc supplementation have been reported with modest zinc supplementation (Walravens, 1989). A meta-analysis of growth data from various zinc intervention trials have confirmed that there is a widespread occurrence of growth-limiting zinc deficiency in young children, especially in developing countries. Research also indicates that zinc availability affects cell-signaling systems which coordinate the response to the growth-regulating hormone, insulin-like growth factor-1 (IGF-1) (Walravens, 1989; Hambidge, 2000; MacDonald, 2000). Zinc supplementation has been linked with improved motor development in very low-birth-weight infants, more vigor in activity in Indian infants and toddlers, and more functional activity in Guatemalan infants and toddlers (Caulfield, 1998).

Zinc and immune response in the elderly

Age-related reduction in immune function is similar to one associated with zinc deficiency, and the elderly are susceptible to mild zinc deficiency. However, the results of zinc supplementation trials on immune function in the elderly have given mixed results. Certain aspects of immune function in the elderly have been found to improve with zinc supplementation (Salgueiro, 2000). In a randomized placebo-controlled study in men and women above 65 years of age, a zinc supplement of 25 mg/day for three months increased levels of some circulating immune cells (*i.e.*, CD4 T-cells and cytotoxic T-lymphocytes) compared to placebo (Fortes, 1998). However, in other studies zinc supplementation did not improve parameters of immune function, indicating that more research may be required before any recommendations can be made about zinc and immune system response in the elderly.

Zinc and pregnancy complications

It has been anticipated that 82% of pregnant women worldwide are likely to be inadequate in zinc intakes. Poor maternal zinc nutritional status is likely cause of a number of adverse outcomes of pregnancy, including low birth weight, premature delivery, labor, delivery complications, and congenital anomalies (Shah and Sachdev, 2006). However, the maternal zinc supplementation trials in the U.S. and developing countries have not given conclusive results (Caulfield *et al.*, 1998). Some studies have found maternal zinc supplementation to increase the birth weight and decrease the likelihood of premature delivery. But, two placebo-controlled studies in Peruvian and Bangladeshi women found zinc supplementation to be ineffective in the incidence of low birth weight or premature delivery (Caulfield *et al.*, 1999; Osendarp, 2000). Supplementation studies conducted to assess the effect of zinc supplementation on labor and delivery complications have also generated some what mixed results, though only some have been conducted in zinc-deficient populations (Caulfield *et al.*, 1998). A systematic review of 17 randomized controlled trials indicated that zinc supplementation during pregnancy resulted in a 14% reduction in premature deliveries; the lower incidence of preterm births mainly in low-income women. This analysis, however, did not suggest zinc supplementation to be of benefit other indicators of maternal or infant health (Mahomed 2007).

Zinc in disease treatment

A meta-analysis of randomized controlled trials has concluded that zinc supplementation reduced the frequency, severity, and duration of diarrheal episodes in children below five years of age (Aggarwal, 2007). The World Health Organization and the United Nations Children's Fund have recommended zinc supplementation as part of the treatment for diarrheal diseases in young children (UNICEF/WHO, 2004). A pooled analysis of a number of studies in developing countries has demonstrated a considerable reduction in the prevalence of pneumonia in children supplemented with zinc (Bhutta, 1999). Another meta-analysis has found that zinc supplementation reduced the incidence but not duration of pneumonia or respiratory tract illnesses in children under five years of age (Aggarwal, 2007). Due to conflicting reports, it is not yet clear if zinc supplementation has value in treating childhood malaria (Shankar, 2000; Muller *et al.*, 2001; Sazawal *et al.*, 2007) (Plate 21).

Symptoms for which Zinc deficiency has been implicated as a factor

- Birth Defects
- Low Birth Weight
- Delayed Sexual Development
- Impaired Learning
- Loss of Smell and Taste Sensation
- Diminished Wound Healing
- Anorexia
- Loss of Appetite
- Paranoia
- Depression
- Strong Body Odor
- Benign Prostatic Hypertrophy
- Impotence
- Some Hair, Nail and Joint Conditions
- Arthritic Problems
- Cataracts
- Optic Neuritis
- Skin Conditions such as Acne and Dermatitis
- Defective Bone Mineralization
- Weight Loss
- Lack of Sexual Development
- Infections
- Small Breasts in Females
- Growth Retardation
- Dwarfism
- Delayed Puberty in Adolescents
- Rough Skin
- Poor Appetite
- Mental Lethargy
- Short Stature
- Diarrhea
- Pneumonia
- Stretch Marks
- Poor Immune Function
- Reduced Collagen (Connective Tissue)
- Acne
- Cross-linking in Collagen
- Macular Degeneration
- Myopia

Plate 21

The use of zinc lozenges on the day of the onset of cold symptoms, and continued every 2–3 h while awake until symptoms resolve, has been prescribed for reducing the duration of the common cold. While five studies in zinc lozenges reduced the duration of cold symptoms, other five studies found no difference between zinc lozenges and placebo lozenges with respect to the duration or severity of cold symptoms. The evidence for the effectiveness in reducing the duration of common colds seems to be lacking (Jackson, 2000; Prasad, 2000; Turner, 2000).

***Age-related macular degeneration (AMD)*:** It is a degenerative disease of the macula, which is the portion of the retina behind the eye involved with central vision. Zinc may play a role in the development of AMD since zinc is found at high concentrations in the part of the retina affected by AMD, retinal zinc content has been shown to decline with age, and the activities of some zinc-dependent retinal enzymes have been shown to decline with age. However, scientific evidence about zinc intake to be associated with the development or progression of AMD has been limited (Va ndenLangenberg *et al.,* 1998; Smith *et al.,* 1999; Cho *et al.,* 2001; Evans, 2002).

***Diabetes mellitus*:** Moderate zinc deficiency is likely to be relatively common in patients of diabetes mellitus but, whether it is a cause or effect is not known. Zinc supplementation of 50 mg/day had adverse effect on control of blood glucose in insulin-dependent (type 1) diabetics (Cunningham, 1994). In another study, supplementation of type 2 diabetics with 30 mg/day of zinc for six months reduced plasma TBARS but did not significantly affect blood glucose control (Anderson, 2001). Role of zinc on glucose metabolism therefore needs further investigations (King, 2006).

***HIV/AIDS*:** Zinc is considered as essential in maintaining immune system function and HIV-infected individuals are likely to be zinc deficient. In HIV-infected patients, low serum levels of zinc have been found in a more advanced stage of the disease with increased mortality (Lai *et al.,* 2001; Wellinghausen *et al.,* 2000). In AIDS patients, 45 mg/day of zinc for one month resulted in a lowering the incidence of opportunistic infections compared to placebo (Mocchegiani and Muzzioli, 2000). However, since the HIV virus itself requires zinc, excessive zinc intake can stimulate the progression of HIV infection. These results suggest need for further research to determine optimal zinc intakes for HIV-infected individuals (Baum *et al.,* 2000; Kupka and Fawzi, 2002).

Food sources of zinc: Shellfish, beef, and other red meats are rich sources for both total zinc content and zinc bioavailability (the fraction of zinc retained and used by the body). This is because of the relative absence of compounds that inhibit zinc absorption and the presence of certain amino acids (cysteine and methionine) for absorption (King *et al.*, 2006). Nuts and legumes are promising good plant sources of zinc. However zinc in whole grain products and plant proteins is less bioavailable due to high content of phytic acid, which inhibits zinc absorption. The enzymatic action of yeast reduces the level of phytic acid in foods. Therefore, fermented whole grain breads have more bioavailable zinc than unfermented whole grain breads.

The incidences of acute zinc toxicity have occurred due to consumption of food or beverages contaminated with zinc released from galvanized containers. Signs of acute zinc toxicity are abdominal pain, diarrhea, nausea, and vomiting. Single doses of 225 to 450 mg of zinc usually induce vomiting. Milder gastrointestinal distress has been reported at doses of 50 to 150 mg/day of supplemental zinc. Metal fume fever has been reported after the inhalation of zinc oxide fumes. Specifically, profuse sweating, weakness, and rapid breathing may develop within eight hours of zinc oxide inhalation and persists 12-24 hours after exposure is terminated (FNB, 2001; King *et al.,* 2006).

Some recent reports on zinc nutrition

Zinc and NCDs

Oxidative stress and chronic inflammation have been linked with development of many cancers. In patients with head and neck cancer, nearly 65% were zinc deficient based on their cellular zinc levels. Natural killer (NK) cell activity and IL-2 generation also had effect but adversely. Th2 cytokines were not affected. Among patients, zinc status was a better indicator of tumor load and stage of disease in comparison to the overall nutritional status. Zinc status was correlated with a number of hospital admissions and incidences of infections. NF-kappa B is constitutively activated in many cancer cells, and resulting in activation of antiapoptotic genes, VEGF, cyclin DI, EGFR, MMP-9 and inflammatory cytokines (Prasad *et al.,* 2009).

Zinc is necessary in the metabolism of melatonin. Hence, it can be a very important factor in the treatment of attention deficit and hyperactivity disorder (ADHD). A study of ADHD treatment with zinc sulfate as a supplement to methylphenidate showed beneficial effects of zinc supplementation for treating children with ADHD. The dose of zinc sulfate (55 mg/day), was equivalent to 15 mg zinc (Dodig-Curkoviæ, 2009).

Zinc deficiency seems to be a major factor underlying taste impairment and A po/no 10 activities of angiotensin converting enzyme. (ACE ratio) may predict the prognosis for taste impairment after zinc supplementation, and to be a more sensitive indicator of zinc nutrition, rather than zinc concentration in the serum (Takaoka *et al.,* 2010).

In the Western Highlands of Guatemala, 412 infants randomly received low-phytate or control maize. Within each maize group, infants were further randomly grouped to receive a zinc supplement or placebo. Low linear growth in older Guatemalan infants did not improve with both the low-phytate maize and a daily 5-mg zinc supplement (Mazariegos *et al.*, 2010).

In developing countries, zinc supplementation may be beneficial for the prevention of upper respiratory infection and diarrhea, and as complementary therapy for diarrhea in malnourished children. Zinc coupled with antioxidants may be modestly effective in retarding the progression of intermediate and advanced age-related macular degeneration. Zinc has been effective treatment also for Wilson disease (Saper and Rash, 2009).

Zinc deficiency is the cause of dysfunction of humoral and cell-mediated immunity and increases the susceptibility to infection. Supplementation of zinc reduced the incidence of infection as well as cellular damage from increased oxidative stress. Zinc deficiency has been also associated with acute and chronic liver disease. Zinc supplementation protects against toxin-induced liver damage and in use as a therapy for hepatic encephalopathy in patients that are refractory to standard treatment (Tuerk and Fazel, 2009).

Clinical studies revealed that depression is accompanied by low serum zinc, which can be normalized by successful antidepressant treatment. Moreover, a preliminary clinical study demonstrated the beneficial effect of zinc supplementation as antidepressant therapy in treatment for non-resistant and resistant patients (Szewczyk *et al.*, 2010).

The average Cd was increased, while level of Zn was decreased in the blood and scalp hair samples of mouth cancer patients as compared to referent subjects ($p<.001$) (Kazi *et al.*, 2010). Twenty-six patients with subacute stroke, were randomly divided to a control group (n=13) or Zn^{2+} group (n=13) of 10 mg Zn^{2+}/day. Neurological gravity was measured with the NIH stroke scale (NIHSS) at time of patient admission and after 30 days of protocol period. At day 30, the improvement in NIHSS was significantly higher in the zinc group than in the placebo (-4.7 +/- 1.3 points versus -3.3 +/- 1.1 points; $p<0.02$). Further, NIHSS and Zn^{2+} intake were negatively correlated ($r = -0.46$; $p<0.02$) (Aquilani *et al.*, 2009).

The impact of trace metal deficiencies on the early stages of atherosclerosis has not been well studied in patients with chronic kidney disease CKD and in obese people, although the influence of trace elements depletion, particularly zinc (Zn), may have significant clinical implications. A brief review has described the functions of Zn as well as its in atherosclerosis processes, with a particular emphasis on obese patients with CKD (Lobo *et al.,* 2009).

Zinc deficiency is known to occur in widely diverse states, like ESRD patients on maintenance hemodialysis (HD). A sub normal level of the serum total cholesterol was a factor associated with malnutrition and morbidity in the HD patients. Maintenance HD patients with both low serum zinc and low serum total cholesterol may benefit by zinc supplementation (Roozbeh *et al.,* 2009).

Erythrocyte zinc was significantly lower in chronic pancreatitis patients than that in the controls (26.5+/-9.5 microg/g Hb *vs.* 38.0+/-6.6 microg/g Hb; p<0.001), and in tropical chronic pancreatitis than in alcoholic chronic pancreatitis (25.0+/-10.4 microg/g Hb *vs.* 29.6+/-6.5 microg/g Hb, p=0.001). In chronic pancreatitis patients having exocrine insufficiency, erythrocyte zinc positively correlated with stool elastase1 (r=0.587, p<0.001). Erythrocyte zinc was significantly lower in diabetic patients as compared to non-diabetics (p=0.036). This study demonstrated zinc deficiency in chronic pancreatitis patients, and also its association with exocrine and endocrine insufficiency (Girish *et al.,* 2009).

Review of the existing literature suggests associations between micronutrient deficiencies and obesity in different populations. These associations and possible mechanisms of the deficiencies' metabolic effects, such as their influence on leptin and insulin metabolism, have been discussed. It has been concluded that further studies are needed to clarify the roles of the different micronutrient deficiencies with respect to obesity and its comorbid conditions (Garcia *et al.,* 2009).

Zinc for children

Severe zinc deficiency in children can cause a fatal condition called acrodermatitis enteropathica. The same syndrome has been also observed in patients on total parenteral nutrition (TPN) who have not received zinc. In TPN, Zn requirements have been estimated by balance studies to be 3 mg/d in patients without gastrointestinal losses and a 12 mg/d in patients with diarrhea and fistula losses (Jeejeebhoy, 2009).

A total of, 609 children were followed up for 120 days for information on morbidity of which, 73.3% were zinc-deficient (plasma zinc < 70 microg/dL), and 33.8% had levels of plasma zinc below 60 microg/dL. A significantly higher risk of morbidity was prevalent among the children with lower plasma zinc as compared to those with higher levels of plasma zinc (Dhingra *et al.,* 2009).

Prenatal iron-zinc supplementation was found to increase the mean birthweight for anaemic and iron-deficient women but not for women with higher iron stores in early pregnancy (Saaka *et al.,* 2009).

Beneficial therapeutic response of zinc supplementation has been reported for the diarrhea of children, chronic hepatitis C, shigellosis, leprosy, tuberculosis, pneumonia, acute lower respiratory tract infection, common cold, and leishmaniasis. Zinc supplementation was useful in reducing incidences of infections in the elderly, in patients with sickle cell disease (SCD) and lower in a incidences of respiratory tract infections in children. Zinc supplementation had prevented blindness for 25% of the elderly individuals with dry type of AMD. It was also effective in reducing oxidative stress and generation of inflammatory cytokines such as TNF-alpha and IL-1beta in elderly individuals and patients with SCD (Prasad, 2009). Children with chronic liver disease, both a compensated or decompensated state, had lower serum zinc compared with the healthy controls. As the severity of liver disease increased, the zinc levels decreased. The study suggested that zinc supplementation should form part of the micronutrient intake of children with chronic liver disease (Umusig-Quitain and Gregorio, 2010).

Zinc and infections

Iron-zinc supplementation lowered the risk of increase in malaria parasitaemia which was associated with high maternal serum ferritin and Hb levels. It was also associated with reduced malaria parasite densities, $F (1, 20) = 4.744$, $p = 0.042$. Iron and zinc provided in the ratio of 1:1 prevented a significant lowering in maternal iron stores of pregnant women. Adjusted geometric mean serum ferritin levels in the Iron-zinc group was significantly higher than in the Control Group (22.9 *vs* 16.9 microg/L), $F (1, 156) = 6.336$, $p = 0.013$ (Saaka *et al.,* 2009).

A significant increase in total-Mg^{2+} saliva concentration, as well as a decrease in Zn^{2+}/Cu^{2+} serum ratio could be considered as a marker for predisposition to oro-maxillar suppurations (Luca *et al.,* 2009).

In vitro models for zinc interactions

A decrease in zinc increases the production of cell oxidants, affects the oxidant defense system and triggers oxidant sensitive signals in neuronal cells. Results by Aimo *et al.* (2010) demonstrate that a decrease in extracellular Zn leads to an increase in neuronal oxidants through the activation of the NMDAR that leads to calcium influx and to a calcium-mediated activation of protein kinase C/NADPH oxidase and NOS. Changes in extracellular Zn concentrations can be sensed by neurons, which using reactive oxygen and nitrogen species as second messengers, can regulate signaling involved in neuronal development and function (Aimo *et al.,* 2010).

A lowering of neuronal zinc can cause cell cycle arrest, which in part involves a deregulation of select signals (ERK1/2, p 53, and NF-kappaB). Zinc deficiency can also induce apoptotic neuronal death through the intrinsic (mitochondrial) pathway, which can be induced by the activation of the zinc-regulated enzyme caspase-3, and as a result of abnormal regulation of prosurvival signals (ERK1/2 and NF-kappaB). Alterations in such finely tuned processes of neurogenesis, neuronal migration, differentiation, and apoptosis, which involve the developmental shaping of the nervous system, could have a long-term consequences on brain health (Adamo and Oteiza, 2010).

Breaking of the intestinal barrier is a causative factor in the development of alcoholic endotoxemia and hepatitis. Caco-2 cell culture demonstrated that alcohol exposure increases the intracellular free zinc due to oxidative stress. Zinc deficiency resulted epithelial barrier disruption in association with disassembling of tight junction proteins in the Caco-2 cells (Zhong *et al.,* 2010).

Zinc is known as an essential nutritional factor in human and animal growth. Bone growth retardation is a common feature of various conditions associated with dietary zinc deficiency. Bone zinc has been shown to decrease in aging, skeletal unloading, and postmenopausal conditions, suggesting its role in bone disorder. Zinc demonstrated enhancing effect on osteoblastic bone formation and mineralization; the metal directly activates aminoacyl-tRNA synthetase, a rate-limiting enzyme at translational process of protein synthesis, in the cells, and it also stimulates cellular protein synthesis (Yamaguchi, 2009).

In vivo models for zinc interactions

Zinc functions in antioxidant defense and DNA repair and could be important factor for prostate health. The study using rats has suggested that marginal zinc deficiency sensitizes the prostate to oxidative stress and demonstrate the importance of maintaining optimal zinc nutrition in physically active populations (Song *et al.*, 2010).

Novel Biological Functions and Interactions of Zinc (Author's Experiments)

1. Interaction of vitamins with zinc using cell and protein models

***Effect of zinc on enterocyte metabolism under normal and oxidative stress conditions*:** Using Caco-2 cells, interactions of folic acid (FA), nicotinic acid (NA), ascorbic acid (AA), riboflavin, thiamine, pyridoxine on intestinal Zn transport and their implications under oxidative stress (OS) conditions were investigated. Without OS, Zn transport was slightly enhanced in presence of NA, while significantly reduced by thiamine, riboflavin and pyridoxine. Under OS, NA increased transport in dose dependent manner. Under both conditions, Zn transport was reduced by FA and not by AA. The levels of catalase, SOD and GPx and OS markers (DCF-DA and tetramethyl rhodamine) varied significantly. Results for the first time demonstrate advantageous effects of NA and deleterious consequences of AA and FA treatments (Tupe and Agte, 2009).

***Antiglycation activity of zinc with glucose as glycating agent and BSA as protein model*:** Long term glycation of circulating proteins like albumin represents consequences of chronic hyperglycemia. Role of Zn alone and in presence of ascorbic acid (AA) and folic acid (FA) in albumin (BSA) glycation performed by incubations of BSA with glucose at 37°C along with Zn, AA, FA separately and as Zn+AA, Zn+FA for 150 days was investigated. Zn inhibited glycation and β aggregation, probably due to observed higher protein bound Zn. It also protected protein thiols and increased cell survival. Both, AA and FA enhanced glycation which was lowered in samples coincubated with Zn. FA increased albumin bound Zn and showed maximum cell survival. These results indicated a new dimension of the role of Zn in hyperglycemic conditions and also helped to understand the interplay of Zn with micronutrients in albumin glycation (Tupe and Agte, 2009).

***Effect of zinc on hepatocyte metabolism under normal and oxidative stress conditions*:** Zinc plays a dual role, as an integral part of metabolic machinery and in protection against reactive oxygen species. Liver is a important site for zinc metabolism for synthesis of zinc metalloproteins and maintaining its homeostasis. However, the factors influencing post absorptive zinc metabolism under normal and oxidative stress (OS) conditions are still not understood. Using rat liver slices, four *in vitro* zinc uptake experiments were conducted to study influence of ascorbic acid and folic acid in normal and oxidative stress conditions with Zn levels representing deficient to excess states (7.7–30.7 millimole/L). Zinc uptakes under OS for four zinc levels were lower than those under normal conditions. Folic acid had significant inhibitory effect on zinc uptake under normal as well as OS conditions in a dose response manner. Nevertheless, dose response of ascorbic acid at four zinc levels indicated its marked enhancing effect under OS condition. Results suggest that folic acid causes inhibitory effect, while ascorbic acid may be protective in OS on liver zinc uptake (Tupe *et al.*, 2007).

***Effect of different dietary zinc levels on hepatic antioxidant and micronutrients indices under oxidative stress conditions*:** Variation in body zinc status may affect levels of riboflavin, niacin and vitamin C in liver, both in presence and absence of oxidative stress (OS). Experiment was carried on weanling male Wistar rats for three weeks. Rats (n=48) were randomly divided into six groups (n=8); 3 levels of dietary zinc; Zn deficient (ZnD, 8 mg/kg diet), Zn normal (ZnN, 30 mg/kg diet) and Zn excess (ZnE, 60 mg/kg diet) with OS present (+OS) and absent (-OS) induced by intra peritoneal injection of tertiary butyl hydro peroxide (t-BHP) at the dose of 0.2 mM/Kg body weight. GPT and GOT showed decreasing trend from ZnD to ZnE irrespective of OS indicating protective effect of zinc. TBARS were significantly lowered while catalase levels were significantly higher in ZnE groups than the other two groups. Liver niacin significantly increased from ZnD to ZnE under both, +OS and –OS groups, whereas in all +OS groups liver niacin was higher than respective –OS groups. Zinc has emerged as protective factor for liver function. Liver zinc, liver niacin and OS have shown complex interrelationship with each other (Tupe *et al.*, 2010).

***Vitamin-zinc interactions in human erythrocytes*:** *In vitro* zinc uptake by human erythrocytes was observed under a range of zinc levels these represent three different plasma zinc levels *i.e.*, zinc deficient [0.35–0.61 ppm], zinc normal [0.74–1.59 ppm], and zinc excess [1.65–2.3 ppm]. Further, interactions of physiological levels of riboflavin, flavin adenine dinucleotide (FAD), nicotinic acid, nicotinamide adenine dinucleotide (NAD), thiamine, thiamine pyrophosphate (TPP), folic acid, and ascorbic acid with zinc uptakes were studied in separate experiments. In control flasks, as compared to the normal zinc state, the rate of change of zinc uptake over change in zinc levels was 1.6 times in the excess state and 0.12 times in the deficient state, indicating three distinct patterns. Under the simulated zinc-deficient state, thiamine significantly enhanced the zinc uptakes ($p<0.05$), but ascorbic acid and riboflavin inhibited zinc uptakes ($p<0.05$). The percent hemolysis of the cells was also significantly lower in the presence of thiamine ($p<0.05$) (Agte *et al.,* 2004).

2. Zinc in health and disease

***Comparative in vitro uptake of zinc by erythrocytes of normal vs Type 2 diabetic individuals was associated with osmotic fragility of erythrocytes*:** Diabetes is an oxidative stress-related disorder in which erythrocyte zinc uptake is likely to be different from healthy individuals. *In vitro* zinc uptake, osmotic fragility and glucose uptake, were compared in Type 2 diabetic subjects (n=43) and healthy controls (n=22). %hemolysis at 0.75, 0.65 and 0.55% NaCl had significant negative associations ($p<0.05$) with *in vitro* zinc uptakes. Further, erythrocyte super oxide dismutase (SOD), plasma ascorbic acid and status of riboflavin and thiamine had negative correlations with *in vitro* zinc uptakes of erythrocytes in healthy subjects ($p<0.01$). The magnitude of associations in the diabetic subjects were lower than normal subjects. Erythrocyte zinc uptake and osmotic fragility could be biomarkers of long-term zinc status and lowering of zinc uptake may be one of the features of diabetic patients (Agte *et al.,* 2004) (Plate 22).

Study of factors affecting binding of zinc with albumin at physiological zinc concentrations: Albumin is known to have very high affinity for many organic and inorganic compounds which influence albumin bound Zn (ABZn). To understand of these molecular interactions, the effects of riboflavin, nicotinic acid, thiamine, folic acid, pyruvic acid and glucose on ABZn were studied. The ABZn was separated from the unbound zinc using equilibrium dialysis and measured by atomic absorption spectrometer. At therapeutic zinc levels, folic acid and thiamine significantly enhanced the ABZn ($p<0.010$), while nicotinic acid inhibited zinc binding to albumin. Folic acid enhanced the ABZn also at lower zinc concentrations representing physiological levels of plasma zinc (138–150 micromoles) ($p<0.05$) (Agte and Nagmote, 2004).

***Effect of vitamin supplementation on zinc and iron absorption*:** Diets prevalent in vegetarian populations with rice and other whole grains and with little consumption of yellow vegetables are low in riboflavin. Experiments were conducted on two groups each of 12 pregnant and lactating mice (9 females and 3 males on a low-riboflavin rice-based diet with and one without supplementation of 10 mg riboflavin/kg diet. There was significant improvement in the growth parameters like % conception, mean weight gain in pregnancy, mean weight of pups at the age of 21 d, and % hemoglobin due to riboflavin supplementation ($p<0.05$). Percent zinc absorption, for the low-riboflavin diet, the supplemented diet, and the synthetic control diet were 16.4 ± 5.7, 33.7 ± 8.9, and 44.6 ± 4.0, respectively, indicating the enhancing effect of riboflavin supplementation on iron and zinc utilization (Agte *et al.,* 1998).

***Interaction of nicotinic acid with zinc metabolism*:** Nicotinic acid has functional groups that can form complexes with trace metals. The effect of nicotinic acid supplementation on absorption and utilization of zinc and iron was studied, *in vitro* zinc uptake by human erythrocytes of 10 healthy subjects. It was increased by 38.9% and 43.1% in fasting, and by 70.9% and 28.1% in postprandial conditions with 8 mumoles nicotinic acid or NADP. The results of animal experiments suggested that nicotinic acid, in addition to its known effect on growth and metabolism, may be also playing a role in enhancing zinc and iron utilization (Agte *et al.,* 1997).

***Bioavailability of zinc and other micronutrients in human ileostomy model*:** Apparent absorption of eight micronutrients and degradation of phytic acid were studied in human subjects ileostomised. Percentage of absorption for ascorbic acid showed weak positive associations with intakes of riboflavin ($r=0.71$) and ascorbic acid ($r=0.5$). Percentage of absorption of ascorbic acid was positively correlated with % of absorption of β-carotene ($r=0.80$, $P<0.05$), iron, and riboflavin ($r=0.64$, $P=0.086$), indicating some common influencing factors. Percentages of absorption for zinc (20.2), iron (9.9), and copper (17.6) were comparable with those reported for soy protein-based, high phytate diets. Pattern of phytic acid in the meals and output indicated partial degradation and absorption (34%). For vegetarian Indian meals, apparent absorptions of β-carotene and ascorbic acid were 76% and 73.5% and of riboflavin and thiamine was 63%. Zinc, copper, and iron showed a lower absorption of 10% to 20% (Agte *et al.,* 2005) (Plate 22).

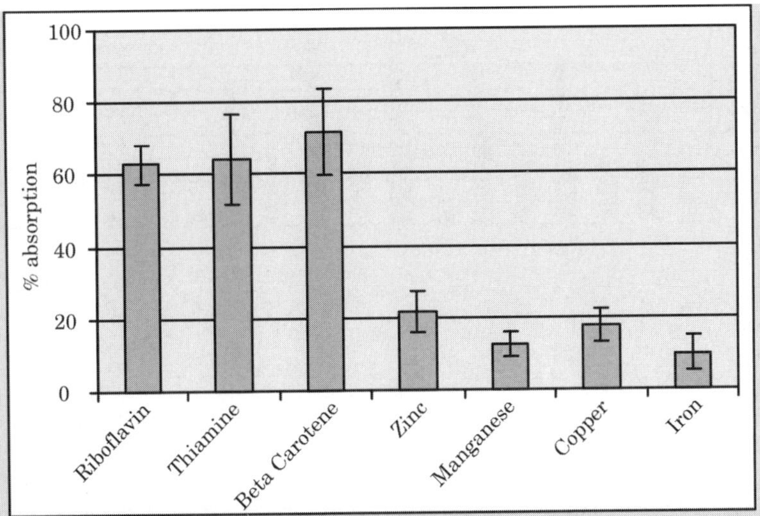

Average absorption of micronutrients from vegetarian meals in 8 ileostomy patients (Agte *et al* 2005)

Plate 22

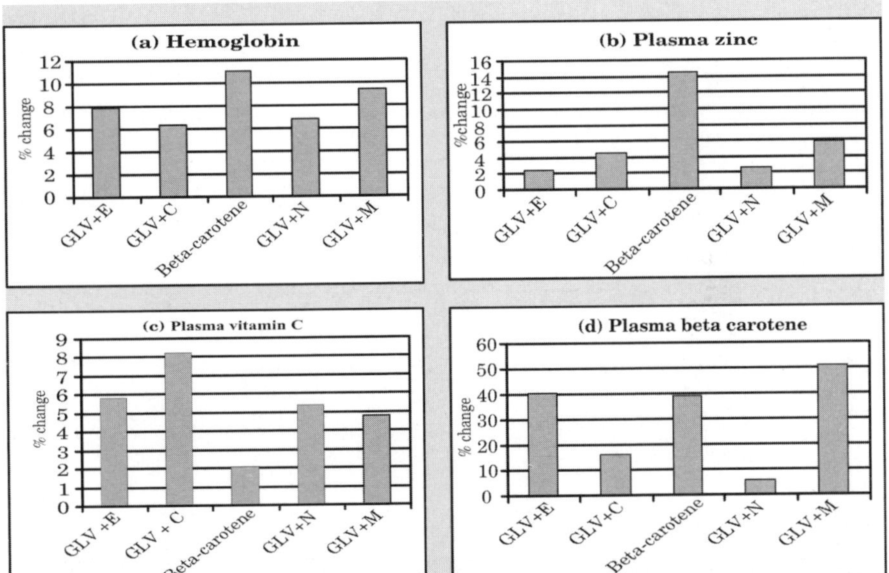

Three weeks' Green Leafy Vegetables supplements increased micronutrient status in young adults (Agte *et al*, EJN 2005).

Plate 23

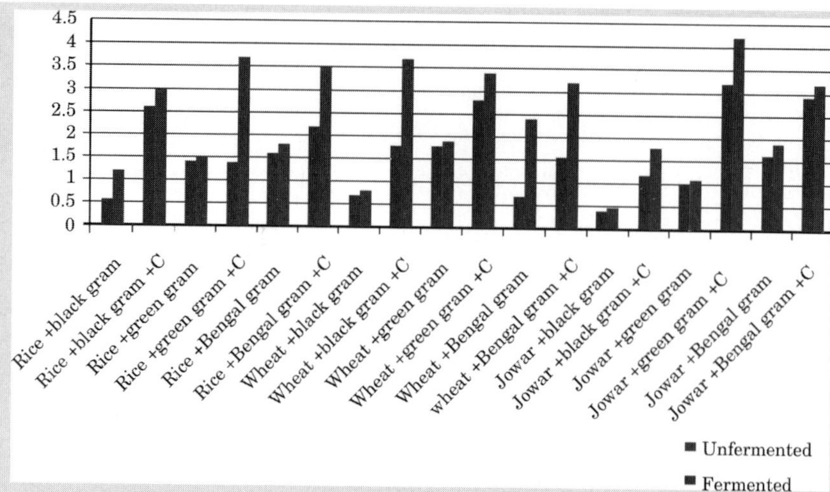

Effect of fermentation and addition of coriander on ionisable iron (mg/100g) in different cereal and legume combinations (Agte and Indumadhavi, 1992)

Plate 24

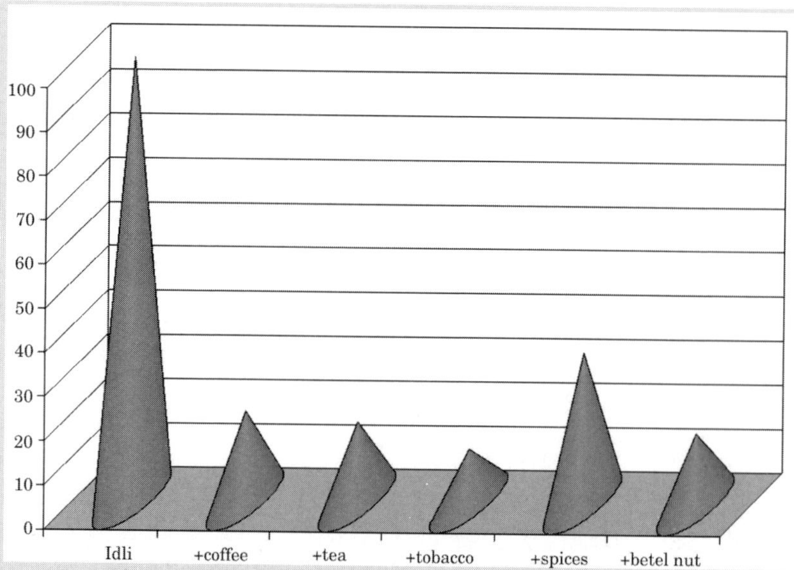

V.V. Agte, M. Indumadhavi., V. Kakade, K.V. Tarwadi, S.A. Chiplonkar. Role of diet related habits and cooking practices on bio availabiltiy of iron, copper and zinc and status of iron in vegetarians. TEMA10, 2000

Effects of habits on total bioavailable Fe as % of Idli

Plate 25

Keeping the wheat flour batter in refrigerator for 12 hours prior to chapatti making enhances zinc solubility by 38.5% due to degradation of phytic acid by 40% (Agte and Joshi, 1997)

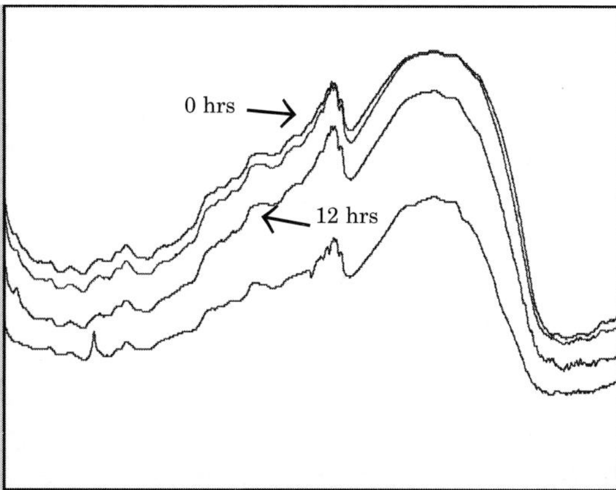

Gradient elution ion exchange chromatography indicated degradation of phytate esters

Effect of traditional processing on phytate degradation in wheat and millets

Plate 26

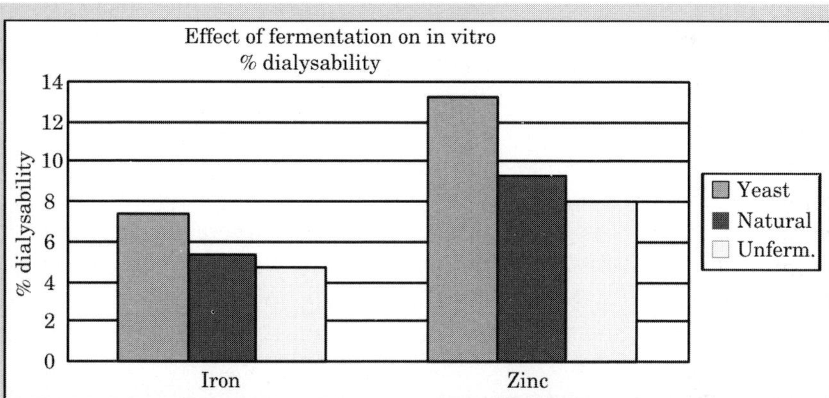

Strategies for improving bioavailable amounts of iron and zinc from vegetarian meals: yeast fermentation and addition of legumes (Agte *et al.*, 1999)

Plate 27

***Prediction of bioavailable zinc from lower phytate forms, folic acid and their interactions with zinc in vegetarian meals*:** A database on *in vitro* zinc dialysability (by isotopic tracer, ^{65}Zn) of vegetarian meals from Asia, Africa, Europe/US and Latin America has been used to develop a model for estimating zinc bioavailability. Folic acid, IP3 and IP5 were significant factors for bioavailable zinc. Weighted multiple regression equation was: ln (bioavailable zinc in mg) = $-1.701 + 1.285 \times \ln[(\text{IP5 in mg}) \times (\text{Zn in mg})] - 1.222 \times \ln(\text{IP5 in mg}) - 0.0078 \times$

folic acid in µg –0.137 × ln [(IP3 in mg) × (Zn in mg)] with adjusted R^2 = 0.64, p = 0.0001 (Chiplonkar and Agte, 2006).

GLV supplements increased plasma β–carotene, vitamin C, zinc and hemoglobin in young healthy adults: Green leafy vegetables (GLV) are rich sources of β–carotene, iron and other micronutrients. The effect of GLV as a natural fortificant of multiple micronutrients through a prospective human trial was investigated through 3 weeks' supplementation in 5 groups of young adults (n=40) given either 100 g GLV/day alone or with tablets of vitamin E (100 mg/day), or C (100 mg/day) or more oil (5 g/day) or non–GLV meal with tablet of β–carotene (10 mg/day). GLV with more oil showed in significant increase of plasma β–carotene (51%) and Hb (9%). GLV with vitamin E had a significant increase in plasma β–carotene (40%), Hb (8%) and plasma vitamin C (6%). Supplementing β–carotene without GLV significantly increased Hb (11%), plasma zinc (14%) in addition to β–carotene. Multiple regression analyses weighted for energy intake indicated a significant association of % increase in Hb with intakes of iron, riboflavin, folic acid, β–carotene, copper, phytate and fiber ($p<0.01$), % change in plasma zinc with intakes of zinc, β–carotene, vitamin C, riboflavin, copper, iron, and thiamin ($p<0.01$), % change in vitamin C with intakes of vitamin C, vitamin E, niacin, riboflavin, thiamin, β–carotene, zinc, phytate and fiber ($p<0.05$) and % change in plasma β–carotene with intakes of β–carotene, thiamin, folic acid, zinc, phytate and tannins ($p<0.05$). Using 100 g GLV/day with 10 g oil could be a single moderate strategy for supplementation of iron, β–carotene, ascorbic acid and zinc (Agte *et al.*, 2006).

AN OVERVIEW OF MINERALS

Calcium

Calcium is the major inorganic element in the human body. About 99% of the calcium in the body is found in bones and teeth, while the remaining 1% is found in the blood and soft tissue. Calcium levels in the blood and fluid surrounding the cells (extracellular fluid) need to be maintained within a very narrow concentration range for normal physiological functioning. The physiological functions of calcium are so vital to survival that, the body will demineralize bone to maintain normal blood calcium levels when calcium intake is inadequate. Thus, adequate dietary calcium is a critical factor in maintaining a healthy skeleton (Weaver *et al.,* 1999) (Table 3.10).

Table 3.10: Calcium at a glance

Name and food sources	***Biological function***	***Preventive role in diseases***	***Toxic effects***	***RDA***
Calcium Milk and milk products, beans, green leafy vegetables	Formation of bones and teeth. Blood clotting, the constriction and relaxation of blood vessels, nerve impulse transmission, muscle contraction, and the secretion of insulin. Excitable cells, such as skeletal muscle and nerve cells, contain voltage-dependent calcium channels in their membranes.	Osteoporosis Pregnancy-induced hypertension (PIH) High blood pressure (hypertension) Premenstrual Syndrome, May lower the risk of colon cancer, Lead toxicity, may also help to induce sleep.	Role in kidney stone formation is controversial.	1,000 mg-1,500 mg/day for adults.

Chromium

The trivalent chromium has been accepted as a nutritionally essential mineral, but it not yet well known exactly how it functions in the body. The two most common forms of chromium are trivalent chromium (III) and hexavalent chromium (VI). Chromium (III) is the principal form in foods as well as the form utilized by the body. Chromium (VI) is derived from chromium (III) by heating at alkaline pH and is used as a source of chromium for industrial purposes. It is a strong irritant and is recognized as a carcinogen when inhaled. At low levels, chromium (VI) is readily reduced to chromium (III) by reducing substances in foods and the acidic environment of the stomach, which serve to prevent the ingestion of chromium (VI) (FNB, 2001, Lukaski, 1999; Stoecker, 1999).

Table 3.11: Chromium at a glance

Name food and sources	***Biological function***	***Preventive role in diseases***	***Toxic effects***	***RDA***
Chromium Grapes, orange, banana, apple, potato, beans, Animal foods	Glucose tolerance factor, insulin requires chromium to function	Diabetes, increases lean body mass and decreases body fat may show reductions in serum total cholesterol, LDL-cholesterol, and triglyceride levels or increases in HDL-cholesterol levels increasing the risk for heart disease	Human carcinogen at a high enough dose regardless of the formulation as metal can accumulate in tissues over years	50-200-mcg day for adults

Copper

In the body, copper shifts between the cuprous (Cu^{1+}) and cupric (Cu^{2+}) forms, though the majority of the body's copper is in the Cu^{2+} form. The ability of copper to easily accept and donate electrons explains its important role in oxidation-reduction (redox) reactions and in scavenging free radicals (Linder and Hazegh-Azam, 1996). Although Hippocrates is said to have prescribed copper compounds to treat diseases as early as 400 B.C. (Turnlund, 2006), scientists are still uncovering new information regarding the functions of copper in the human body.

Table 3.5: Copper at a glance

Name food and source	*Biological*	*Preventive role function*	*Toxic in diseases*	*RDA effects*
Copper Animal foods, nuts, oilseeds GLVs	Component of cytochrome c oxidase, role in cellular energy production, lysyl oxidase, cross-linking of collagen and elastin ceruloplasmin (ferroxidase I) and ferroxidase II to oxidize ferrous iron to ferric iron loaded as transferrin, for red blood cell formation, function of the brain and nervous system through Dopamine—mono oxygenase, Monoamine oxidase, myelin synthesis depends on cytochrome c oxidase activity, tyrosinase, formation of melanin pigment of the hair, skin, and eyes, Superoxide dismutase catalyzing the conversion of superoxide radicals hydrogen peroxide, Ceruloplasmin functions as an antioxidant, regulation specific genes transcription.	Copper deficiency leads to anemia, abnormally low numbers of white blood cells known as neutrophils may be accompanied by increased susceptibility to infection. Osteoporosis, loss of pigmentation, neurological symptoms, and impaired growth.	The tolerable upper level of intake (UL) for copper at 10 mg/ day from food and supple-ments.	Adult men and women ages 19 years and older: 900 mcg/day.

Fluorine

Fluorine occurs naturally as the fluoride ion (F^-) and considered as a trace element because only small amounts are present in the body (about 2.6 grams in adults), and because the daily requirement for maintaining dental health is only a few milligrams a day. About 95% of the total body fluoride is found in bones and teeth. Its role in the prevention of dental caries (tooth decay) is well established, but, fluoride is not generally considered an essential mineral element for humans which is required for growth or to sustain life. However, if one considers the prevention of chronic disease (dental caries) an important criterion in determining essentiality, then fluoride might well be considered an essential trace element (Higdon, 2001) (Table 3.12).

Table 3.12: Flourine at a glance

Name food and sources	*Biological function*	*Preventive role in diseases*	*Toxic effects*	*RDA*
Flourine	As fluoroapatite it hardens tooth enamel and stabilizes bone mineral.	Inadequate fluoride intake is an increased risk of dental caries (tooth decay)	Moderate dental fluorosis is characterized by mottling and mild staining of the teeth, and severe dental fluorosis results in marked staining and pitting of the teeth. In its moderate to severe forms, dental fluorosis becomes a cosmetic concern when it affects the incisors and canines (front teeth).	Infants 0.5 mg/ day Children 0.7-2 mg/day Adults 3 mg/ day.

Iodine

Iodine, a non-metallic trace element, is required by humans for the synthesis of thyroid hormones. Iodine deficiency is an important health problem throughout most of the world. Most of the earth's iodine is found in oceans, and iodine content in the soil varies with region. The older an exposed soil surface, the more likely the iodine has been leached away by erosion. Mountainous regions, such as the Himalayas, the Andes, and the Alps, and flooded river valleys, such as the Ganges, are among the most severely iodine-deficient areas in the world (Hetzel *et al.,* 1999) (Table 3.13).

Magnesium

Magnesium plays important roles in the structure and the function of the human body. The adult human body contains about 25 grams of magnesium. Over 60% of all the magnesium in the body is found in the skeleton, about 27% is found in muscle, 6% to 7% is found in other cells, and less than 1% is found outside of cells (Shils, 1997). Magnesium is involved in more than 300 essential metabolic reactions (Spencer *et al.,* 1994) (Table 3.14).

Table 3.13: Iodine at a glance

Name and food source	*Biological function*	*Preventive role in diseases*	*Toxic effects*	*RDA*
Iodine Sea foods and sea vegetables, cod, haddock, mackerel, iodised table salt, milk, brazil nuts.	Essential component of the thyroid hormones thyroxine (T4) and triiodothy-ronine (T3), which regulate growth, development, metabolism, and reproductive function.	Deficiency may lead to cretinism (congenital hypot-hyroidism) and irreversible mental retardation due to maternal deficiency, thyroid hypertrophy (*i.e.* endemic goiter), predisposing to cancer of thyroid, abnormal brain development and consequently impaired intellectual development in infants. Hypot-hyroidism and varying degrees of other developmental abnormities.	Excessive exposure can cause iododerma, fever, salivary gland enlargement, visual problems Symptoms of acute iodine poisoning include burning of the mouth, throat, and stomach, fever, nausea, vomiting, diarrhea, a weak pulse, and coma, Upper safe limit 500 µg.	Approxim-ately 1 µg per kg of body weight is required. The RDA for adults is 150 µg Infants 110–130 µg Children 90–120 µg.

Table 3.14: Magnesium at a glance

Name & sources	*Biological*	*Preventive role function*	*Toxic in diseases*	*RDA effects*
Magne-sium Cereal bran, nuts, beans	A mineral that acts as a cofactor for many functions in the body such as helping with energy production in muscle cells and protein synthesis. Magnesium is required for a number of steps during nucleic acid and protein synthesis. Several enzymes participating in the synthesis of carbohydrates and lipids require magnesium for their activity. Glutathione requires magnesium for its synthesis. Magnesium plays a structural role in bone, cell membranes, and chromosomes, required for the active transport potassium and calcium across cell membranes and important in wound healing.	Hypertension (high blood pressure) Preeclampsia-eclampsia (toxemia of pregnancy) Diabetes mellitus Cardiovascular disease Migraine headaches Asthma Osteoporosis.	Elevated levels may result in a fall in blood pressure. Lethargy, confusion, disturbances in normal cardiac rhythm, and deterioration of kidney function.	310–420 mg/day for adults.

Molybdenum

Molybdenum is an essential trace element for virtually all life forms. It functions as a cofactor for a number of enzymes that catalyze important chemical transformations in the global carbon, nitrogen, and sulfur cycles (Wuebbens, 2000). Thus, molybdenum-dependent enzymes are not only required for human health, but also for the health of our ecosystem (Table 3.15).

Table 3.15: Molybdenum at a glance

Name and food sources	*Biological function*	*Preventive role in diseases*	*Toxic effects*	*RDA*
Molybdenum Legumes, such as beans, lentils, and peas, are the richest sources of molybdenum. Grain products and nuts are considered good sources.	The biological form of molybdenum is known as the molybdenum cofactor for three enzymes. Sulfite oxidase, xanthine oxidase and aldehyde oxidase which contributes to the antioxidant capacity of the blood also play a role in the metabolism of drugs and toxins.	Deficiency in TPN results in rapid heart and respiratory rates, headache, night blindness, and ultimately became comatose. Also low blood uric acid levels, decreased urinary excretion of uric acid and sulfate, and increased urinary excretion of sulfite. Molybdenum supplementation (160 mcg/day) reversed the amino acid intolerance and improved the clinical condition.	Increased blood uric acid levels and gout-like symptoms have been reported in occupationally exposed workers consuming 10 to 15 mg of molybdenum from food daily However, a controlled study found no serious adverse effects of molybdenum intakes of up to 1.5 mg/day (1,500 mcg/day) for 24 days in four healthy young men.	45 µg for adult men and women 50 µg for pregnancy and lactation 17–43 µg for 1–18 yrs age.

Potassium

Potassium is an essential dietary mineral which is an electrolyte in nature *viz.* a substance that dissociates into ions (charged particles) in solution, making it capable of conducting electricity. Normal body function depends on tight regulation of potassium concentrations both inside and outside of cells (Peterson, 1997) (Table 3.16).

Table 3.16: Potassium at a glance

Name and food sources	***Biological function***	***Preventive role in diseases***	***Toxic effects***	***RDA***
Potassium Fruits and vegetables nuts, oilseeds, dairy foods and other animal products.	Maintenance of normal water balance, regulation of neuromuscular activity. We need it for normal cell growth. Potassium is related to muscle mass and glucose storage, if muscle is being formed, an adequate supply of potassium is essential.	Potassium seems to be protective against hypertension and may control blood pressure more effectively than a low sodium diet. Potassium helps to make arteries stronger and better able to withstand the blood vessel damage that occurs with aging. Decreased risk of stroke, osteoporosis and kidney stones. Muscle cramps-Electrolyte imbalance such s lack of potassium may play a role in muscle cramps.	Excess potassium causes an increased fibrillation of the heart and death in extreme cases.	4700 mg/day for adults

Phosphorus

Phosphorus is an essential mineral that is required by every cell in the body for normal function (Knochel, 2006). The majority of the phosphorus in the body is found as phosphate (PO_4). Approximately 85% of the body's phosphorus is found in bone (FNB, 1997) (Table 3.17).

Table 3.17: Phosphorus at a glance

Name and food sources	***Biological function***	***Preventive role in diseases and deficiency symptoms***	***Toxic effects***	***RDA***
Phosphorus Cereal grains, nuts, seeds, meat, poultry and fish, eggs, milk products, pulses, cheese, wheat germ, sardines, peanuts, yeast extract, soya beans.	Necessary for normal bone and tooth structure and growth. It is involved in almost all physiological chemical reactions. Phosphorus in combination with calcium helps to support the body structure.	Deficiency uncommon but may result in bone loss and s characterized by weakness, anorexia and pain Supplements can lessen the pain of arthritis.	None	RDA for adults is 1200 mg.

Sodium

Sodium in the form of common salt (sodium chloride) is essential for life. The tight regulation of the body's sodium and chloride concentrations is so important that multiple mechanisms work in concert to control them. Although scientists agree that a minimal amount of salt is required for survival, the health implications of excess salt intake represent an area of continued investigation among scientists, clinicians, and public health experts (Taubes, 1998) (Table 3.18).

Table 3.18: Sodium at a glance

Name and Food sources	***Biological function***	***Preventive role in diseases and deficiency symptoms***	***Toxic effects***	***RDA***
Sodium Salt, shellfish, spirulina, cheese and red or green peppers.	Principal electrolyte of extracellular fluid. Closely involved with body's water balance together with potassium and chloride. Also has a role in acid-alkaline balance. Corrects nerve and muscle function. Crucial for regulating the membrane potential of cells and is involved in active transport across cell membranes, it is pumped out in exchange for potassium. It helps the nerves and muscles function properly.	The body may be depleted of sodium under extreme conditions of sweating or chronic diarrhoea.	Excessive intake of sodium can result in edema and hypertension.	No RDA is defined but a minimum daily requirement for healthy adults is 500 mg. Indians: 1.6 g.

Table 3.19 gives sources of 3 important than elements and the factors affecting their bioavailability. Nonetheless, trace element research has crossed the boundaries of classical inorganic chemistry and has become an important aspect in human health and disease.

Table 3.19: Information about sources and bioavailability of Ca, Zn & Fe

Nutrient	***Rich sources***	***Enhances of absorption***	***Inhibit of absorption***	***Poor sources***
Calcium	Green vegetables, skim milk, cow's milk, beans, nuts	15 min to 1 hr sunshine or vitamin D from fortified milk or cereals.	Low activity, oxalates.	Milk and milk products Cereal flours GLV
Zinc	Nuts, wheatgerm, whole grain products, brewers yeast, meat, eggs, legumes and seeds.	Histidine Citric acid.	Smoking and alcohol, phytates, fiber, Iron.	Refined flours,
Iron	Green leafy vegetables as salad, oysters, yeast, beans, nuts, seeds and cereals.	Vitamin C, vitamin C rich fruits (orange, lemon, guava, amla) and vegetables (cauliflower, capsicum).	Tea, coffee, bran and phytates, tannins.	Refined flours, pumpkin, brinjal like vegetables.

REFERENCES

Adamo A, and Oteiza P 2010. Zinc deficiency and neurodevelopment: The case of neurons. Biofactors. Mar. 23. [Epub ahead of print].

Aggarwal R, Sentz J, and Miller MA 2007. Role of zinc administration in prevention of childhood diarrhoea and respiratory illnesses: a meta-analysis. *Pediatrics* 119(6): 1120–1130.

Agte V, and Nagmote R 2004. Study of factors affecting binding of zinc with albumin at physiological zinc concentrations. *Bio. Factors* 20: 3/139–145.

Agte V, Nagmote R, and Chiplonkar S 2004. Role of vitamin-zinc interactions on in *vitro* zinc uptake by human erythrocytes. *Biological Trace Element Research* 99: 1–3.

Agte V, Nagmote R, and Tarwadi K 2004. Comparative *in vitro* uptake of zinc by erythrocytes of normal *vs* Type 2 diabetic individuals and the associated factors. *Diabetes Nutr. Metab.* 17(6): 343–9.

Agte V, Paknikar K, and Chiplonkar S 1997. Effect of nicotinic acid on zinc and iron metabolism. *Biometals.* 10(4): 271–6.

Agte V, Jahagirdar M, and Chiplonkar S 2006. GLV supplements increased plasma beta-carotene, vitamin C, zinc and hemoglobin in healthy young adults. *Euro. J. Nutr.* 45: 29–36.

Agte VV, Jahagirdar M, and Chiplonkar SA 2005. Absorption of eight micronutrients and phytic acid from vegetarian meals in human ileostomy volunteers. *Nutrition*, 21(6): 678–685.

Aimo L, Cherr G, and Oteiza PI 2010. Low extracellular zinc increases neuronal oxidant production through, NADPH oxidase and nitric oxide synthase activation. *Free Radic Biol. Med.* [Epub ahead of print].

Akcam M 2010. *Helicobacter pylori* and micronutrients. *Indian Pediatr*. 47(2): 119–26.

Altamura S, and Muckenthaler MU 2009. Iron toxicity in diseases of aging: Alzheimer's disease, Parkinson's disease and atherosclerosis. *J. Alzheimers Dis*. 16(4): 879–895.

Anderson RA, Roussel AM, Zouari N, Mahjoub S, Matheau JM, and Kerkeni A 2001. Potential antioxidant effects of zinc and chromium supplementation in people with type 2 diabetes mellitus. *J. Am. Coll. Nutr.* 20(3): 212–218.

Aquilani R, Baiardi P, Scocchi M, Iadarola P, Verri M, Sessarego P, Boschi F, Pasini E, Pastoris O, and Viglio S 2009. Normalization of zinc intake enhances neurological retrieval of patients suffering from ischemic strokes. *Nutr. Neurosci*. 12(5): 219–25.

Arteel GE, Briviba K, and Sies H 1999. Protection against peroxynitrite. *FEBS Lett*. 445(2–3): 226–230.

Ascherio A, Willett WC, Rimm EB, Giovannucci EL, and Stampfer MJ 1994. Dietary iron intake and risk of coronary disease among men. *Circulation*. 89(3): 969–974.

Aschner JL, and Aschner M 2005. Nutritional aspects of manganese homeostasis. *Mol. Aspects Med*. 26(4–5): 353–362.

Aschner M, 2000. Manganese: brain transport and emerging research needs. *Environ Health Perspect*. 108(Suppl 3): 429–432.

Aschner M, and Dorman DC 2006. Manganese: pharmacokinetics and molecular mechanisms of brain uptake. *Toxicol Rev*. 25(3): 147–154.

Baum MK, and Campa A 2006. Role of selenium in HIV/AIDS. *In*: Hatfield DL, Berry MJ, and Gladyshev VN *Eds*. Selenium: Its Molecular Biology and Role in Human Health. 2nd ed. New York: Springer; pp. 299–310.

Baum MK, Miguez-Burbano MJ, Campa A, and Shor-Posner G 2000. Selenium and interleukins in persons infected with human immunodeficiency virus type 1. *J. Infect Dis*. 182(Suppl 1): S69–73.

Baum MK, Shor-Posner G, and Campa A 2000. Zinc status in human immunodeficiency virus infection. *J. Nutr.* 130(5S Suppl): 1421S-1423S.

Beard J 2006. Iron. *In*: Bowman BA, and Russell RM *Eds*. Present Knowledge in Nutrition. 9th ed. Washington, D.C.: ILSI Press; pp. 430–444.

Beard JL 2001. Iron biology in immune function, muscle metabolism and neuronal functioning. *J. Nutr.* 131(2S–2): 568S–579S.

Beard JL, and Dawson HD 1997. Iron. *In*: O'Dell BL, and Sunde RA, *Eds*. Handbook of nutritionally essential minerals. New York: Marcel Dekker, Inc. pp. 275–334.

Beck MA, 2006. Selenium and viral infections. *In*: Hatfield DL, and Berry MJ, and Gladyshev VN *Eds*. Selenium: Its Molecular Biology and Role in Human Health. 2nd ed. New York: Springer; pp. 287–298.

Benarroch EE, 2009. Brain iron homeostasis and neurodegenerative disease. *Neurology*. 72(16): 1436–1440.

Bhutta ZA, Black RE, Brown KH, *et al*. 1999. Prevention of diarrhea and pneumonia by zinc supplementation in children in developing countries: pooled analysis of randomized controlled trials. Zinc Investigators' Collaborative Group. *J. Pediatr*. 135(6): 689–697.

Bianco AC, and Larsen PR 2006. Selenium, deiodinases and endocrine function. *In*: Hatfield DL, Berry MJ, and Gladyshev VN, *Eds*. Selenium: Its Molecular Biology and Role in Human Health. 2nd ed. New York: Springer. pp. 207–219.

Bleys J, Navas-Acien A, and Guallar E 2007. Serum selenium and diabetes in U.S. adults. *Diabetes Care* 30(4): 829–834.

Bouchard M, Laforest F, Vandelac L, Bellinger D, and Mergler D 2007. Hair manganese and hyperactive behaviors: pilot study of school-age children exposed through tap water. *Environ. Health Perspect* 115(1): 122–127.

Bremner I, 1998. Manifestations of copper excess. *Am. J. Clin. Nutr*. 67(5 Suppl): 1069S–1073S.

Brewer GJ, 2009.The risks of copper toxicity contributing to cognitive decline in the aging population and to Alzheimer's disease. *J. Am. Coll. Nutr.* 28(3): 238–42.

Brinkman M, Reulen RC, Kellen E, Buntinx F, and Zeegers MP 2006. Are men with low selenium levels at increased risk of prostate cancer? *Eur. J. Cancer*. 42(15): 2463–2471.

Brody T, 1999. Nutritional Biochemistry. 2nd ed. San Diego: Academic Press.

Brooks JD, Metter EJ, Chan DW, *et al.* 2001. Plasma selenium level before diagnosis and the risk of prostate cancer development. *J. Urol.* 166(6): 2034–2038.

Burbano X, Miguez-Burbano MJ, McCollister K, *et al.* 2002. Impact of a selenium chemoprevention clinical trial on hospital admissions of HIV-infected participants. *HIV Clin. Trials* 3(6): 483–491.

Burk RF, and Levander OA 1999. Selenium. *In*: Shils M, Olson JA, Shike M, and Ross AC, *Eds*. Modern Nutrition in Health and Disease. 9th ed. Baltimore: Williams & Wilkins. pp. 265–276.

Burk RF, Olson GE, and Hill KE 2006. Deletion of selenoprotein P gene in the mouse. *In*: Hatfield DL, Berry MJ, and Gladyshev VN, *Eds*. Selenium: Its Molecular Biology and Role in Human Health. 2nd ed. New York: Springer. pp. 111–122.

Caulfield LE, Zavaleta N, Figueroa A, and Leon Z 1999. Maternal zinc supplementation does not affect size at birth or pregnancy duration in Peru. *J. Nutr*. 129(8): 1563–1568.

Caulfield LE, Zavaleta N, Shankar AH, and Merialdi M 1998. Potential contribution of maternal zinc supplementation during pregnancy to maternal and child survival. *Am. J. Clin. Nutr*. 68(2 Suppl): 499S–508S.

Cerhan JR, Saag KG, Merlino LA, Mikuls TR, and Criswell LA 2003. Antioxidant micronutrients and risk of rheumatoid arthritis in a cohort of older women. *Am J. Epidemiol*. 157(4): 345–54.

Cesur Y, Yordaman N, and Doðan M 2009. Serum insulin-like growth factor-I and insulin-like growth factor binding protein-3 levels in children with zinc deficiency and the effect of zinc supplementation on these parameters. *J. Pediatr Endocrinol Metab*. 22(12): 1137–43.

Chiplonkar Agte V, 2006. Predicting bioavailable zinc from vegetarian meals. *Journal of the American College of Nutrition*, 25(1): 26–33.

Cho E, Stampfer MJ, Seddon JM, *et al.* 2001. Prospective study of zinc intake and the risk of age-related macular degeneration. *Ann. Epidemiol.* 11(5): 328–336.

Combs GF Jr, and Gray WP 1998. Chemopreventive agents: selenium. *Pharmacol Ther.* 79(3): 179–192.

Constans J, Conri C, and Sergeant C 1999. Selenium and HIV infection. *Nutrition* 15(9): 719–720.

Constans J, Delmas-Beauvieux MC, Sergeant C, *et al.* 1996. One-year antioxidant supplementation with beta-carotene or selenium for patients infected with human immunodeficiency virus: a pilot study. *Clin. Infect Dis.* 23(3): 654–656.

Cousins RJ, 2006. Zinc. *In*: Bowman BA, and Russell RM, *Eds*. Present Knowledge in Nutrition. 9th ed, Vol. 1. Washington, D.C.: ILSI Press. 445–457.

Cunningham JJ, Fu A, Mearkle PL, and Brown RG 1994. Hyperzincuria in individuals with insulin-dependent diabetes mellitus: concurrent zinc status and the effect of high-dose zinc supplementation. *Metabolism.* 43(12): 1558–1562.

Davis JM 1998. Methylcyclopentadienyl manganese tricarbonyl: health risk uncertainties and research directions. *Environ Health Perspect.* 106(Suppl 1): 191–201.

Dekker LH, and Villamor E 2010. Zinc supplementation in children is not associated with decreases in hemoglobin concentrations. *J. Nutr.* [Epub ahead of print].

Delmas-Beauvieux MC, Peuchant E, Couchouron A, *et al.* 1996. The enzymatic antioxidant system in blood and glutathione status in human immunodeficiency virus (HIV)-infected patients: effects of supplementation with selenium or beta-carotene. *Am J. Clin. Nutr.* 64(1): 101–107.

Dhingra U, Hiremath G, Menon VP, Dhingra P, Sarkar A, and Sazawal S 2009. Zinc deficiency: descriptive epidemiology and morbidity among preschool children in peri-urban population in Delhi, India. *J. Health Popul. Nutr.* 27(5): 632–9.

Dobson AW, Erikson KM, and Aschner M 2004. Manganese neurotoxicity. *Ann NY Acad Sci.* 1012: 115–128.

Dodig-CurkoviÄ K, Dovhanj J, CurkoviÄ, *et al.* 2009. The role of zinc in the treatment of hyperactivity disorder in children. *Acta Med. Croatica.* 63(4): 307–13.

Duffield-Lillico AJ, Dalkin BL, Reid ME, *et al.* 2003. Selenium supplementation, baseline plasma selenium status and incidence of prostate cancer: an analysis of the complete treatment period of the Nutritional Prevention of Cancer Trial. *BJU Int.* 91(7): 608–612.

EPA Office of Water 2009. Current Drinking Water Standards. Environmental Protection Agency, 2009 [Web page]. Available at: http://www.epa.gov/safewater/mcl.html

Erikson KM, Thompson K, Aschner J, and Aschner M 2007. Manganese neurotoxicity: a focus on the neonate. *Pharmacol Ther.* 113(2): 369–377.

Evans JR 2002. Antioxidant vitamin and mineral supplements for age-related macular degeneration (Cochrane Review). *Cochrane Database Syst Rev.* (1): CD000254.

Fairbanks VF, 1999. Iron in Medicine and Nutrition. *In*: Shils ME, Olson JA, Shike M, and Ross AC, *Eds*. Modern Nutrition in Health and Disease. 9th ed. Philadelphia: Lippincott Williams & Wilkins. 193–221.

Ferré-Huguet N, Martí-Cid R, Schuhmacher M, and Domingo JL 2008. Risk assessment of metals from consuming vegetables, fruits and rice grown on soils irrigated with waters of the Ebro River in Catalonia, Spain. *Biol. Trace Elem. Res.* 123(1–3): 66–79.

Ferré-Huguet Núria, Martí Nadal, Marta Schuhmacher, and José L. Domingo 2009. Human and Ecological Risk Assessment. *An International Journal*, 15(3): 604–623.

Florescu L, Popa G, Bãlãnicã G, and Azoicãi D 2009. Zinc-essential micronutrient for child health and nutrition. *Rev. Med. Chir. Soc. Med. Nat. Iasi*. 113(3): 650–5.

Food and Nutrition Board, Institute of Medicine 1997. Phosphorus. Dietary Reference Intakes: Calcium, Phosphorus, Magnesium, Vitamin D, and Fluoride. Washington D.C.: National Academy Press. pp. 146–189.

Food and Nutrition Board, Institute of Medicine 2001. Chromium. Dietary reference intakes for vitamin A, vitamin K, boron, chromium, copper, iodine, iron, manganese, molybdenum, nickel, silicon, vanadium, and zinc. Washington, D.C.: National Academy Press. pp. 197–223.

Food and Nutrition Board, Institute of Medicine 2001. Copper. Dietary reference intakes for vitamin A, vitamin K, boron, chromium, copper, iodine, iron, manganese, molybdenum, nickel, silicon, vanadium, and zinc. Washington, D.C.: National Academy Press. pp. 224–257.

Food and Nutrition Board, Institute of Medicine 2001. Iron. Dietary reference intakes for vitamin A, vitamin K, boron, chromium, copper, iodine, iron, manganese, molybdenum, nickel, silicon, vanadium, and zinc. Washington D.C.: National Academy Press. pp. 290–393.

Food and Nutrition Board, Institute of Medicine 2001. Zinc. Dietary reference intakes for vitamin A, vitamin K, boron, chromium, copper, iodine, iron, manganese, molybdenum, nickel, silicon, vanadium, and zinc. Washington, D.C.: National Academy Press. pp. 442–501.

Ford ES, 2000. Serum copper concentration and coronary heart disease among US adults. *Am. J. Epidemiol.* 151(12): 1182–1188.

Fortes C, Forastiere F, Agabiti N, *et al.* 1998. The effect of zinc and vitamin A supplementation on immune response in an older population. *J. Am Geriatr Soc.* 46(1): 19–26.

Foster LH, and Sumar S 1997. Selenium in health and disease: a review. *Crit. Rev. Food Sci. Nutr.* 37(3): 211–228.

García OP, Long KZ, and Rosado JL 2009. Impact of micronutrient deficiencies on obesity. *Nutr. Rev.* 67(10): 559–72.

García-Castiñeiras S 2010. Iron, the retina and the lens: a focused review. *Exp. Eye Res.* 90(6): 664–78. Epub 2010 Mar. 15.

Garland M, Morris JS, Stampfer MJ, *et al.* 1995. Prospective study of toenail selenium levels and cancer among women. *J. Natl. Cancer Inst.* 87(7): 497–505.

Girish BN, Rajesh G, Vaidyanathan K, and Balakrishnan V 2009. Zinc status in chronic pancreatitis and its relationship with exocrine and endocrine insufficiency. *JOP* 10(6): 651–6.

Gladyshev VN, 2006. Selenoproteins and selenoproteomes. *In*: Hatfield DL, Berry MJ, and Gladyshev VN, *Eds*. Selenium: Its molecular biology and role in human health. 2nd ed. New York: Springer. 99–114.

Gothankar SS, Jha SK, Lenka P, Tripathi RM, and Puranik VD 2009. Daily intake of manganese by local population around Kylleng Pyndengsohiong Mawthabah (Domiasiat), Meghalaya in India. *Sci. Total Environ.* 407(8): 2868–71.

Hambidge M, and Krebs N 2000. Zinc and growth. *In*: Roussel AM, *Ed.* Trace elements in man and animals 10: Proceedings of the tenth international symposium on trace elements in man and animals. New York: Plenum Press. pp. 977–980.

Han J, Lee JS, Choi D, *et al.* 2009. Manganese (II) induces chemical hypoxia by inhibiting HIF-prolyl hydroxylase: implication in manganese-induced pulmonary inflammation. *Toxicol Appl. Pharmacol.* 235(3): 261–267.

Hardy IJ, Gillanders L, and Hardy G 2008. Is manganese an essential supplement for parenteral nutrition? *Curr. Opin. Clin. Nutr. Metab. Care.* 11(3): 289–296.

Hendler SS, and Rorvik DR *Eds* 2001. PDR for Nutritional Supplements. Montvale: Medical Economics Company, Inc.

Hetzel BS, and Clugston GA 1999. Iodine. *In*: Shils M, Olson JA, Shike M, and Ross AC, *Eds*. Modern Nutrition in Health and Disease. 9th ed. Baltimore: Williams & Wilkins. pp. 253–264.

Higdon J 2001. Flourine: Micronutrient Information Center. Linus Pauling Institute Oregon State University, p. 1.

Hurwitz BE, Klaus JR, Llabre MM, *et al.* 2007. Suppression of human immunodeficiency virus type 1 viral load with selenium supplementation: a randomized controlled trial. *Arch. Intern. Med.* 167(2): 148–154.

Ip C 1998. Lessons from basic research in selenium and cancer prevention. *J. Nutr.* 128(11): 1845–1854.

Jackson JL, Lesho E, and Peterson C 2000. Zinc and the common cold: a meta-analysis revisited. *J. Nutr.* 130(5S Suppl): 1512S–1515S.

Jackson MJ, 2009. Skeletal muscle aging: role of reactive oxygen species. *Crit Care Med.* 37(10 Suppl): S368–71.

Janus J, and Moerschel SK 2010. Evaluation of anemia in children. *Am Fam. Physician.* 81(12): 1462–71.

Jeejeebhoy K, 2009. Zinc: an essential trace element for parenteral nutrition. *Gastroenterology.* 137(5 Suppl): S7–12.

Johnson MA, Fischer JG, and Kays SE 1992. Is copper an antioxidant nutrient? *Crit. Rev. Food Sci. Nutr.* 32(1): 1–31.

Jones AA, DiSilvestro RA, Coleman M, and Wagner TL 1997. Copper supplementation of adult men: effects on blood copper enzyme activities and indicators of cardiovascular disease risk. *Metabolism.* 46(12): 1380–1383.

Kardinaal AF, Kok FJ, Kohlmeier L, *et al.* 1997. Association between toenail selenium and risk of acute myocardial infarction in European men. The EURAMIC Study. European antioxidant myocardial infarction and breast cancer. *Am J. Epidemiol.* 145(4): 373–379.

Kato I, Dnistrian AM, Schwartz M, *et al.* 1999. Iron intake, body iron stores and colorectal cancer risk in women: a nested case-control study. *Int. J. Cancer.* 80(5): 693–698.

Kazi TG, Wadhwa SK, Afridi HI, Kazi N, Kandhro GA, Baig JA, Shah AQ, Kolachi NF, and Khan S 2010. Evaluation of cadmium and zinc in biological samples of tobacco and alcohol user male mouth cancer patients. *Hum Exp. Toxicol.* 29(3): 221–30.

Keen CL, Ensunsa JL, Watson MH, *et al.* 1999. Nutritional aspects of manganese from experimental studies. *Neurotoxicology* 20(2–3): 213–223.

Kies C, 1994. Bioavailability of manganese. *In*: Klimis-Tavantzis DL, *Ed.* Manganese in health and disease. Boca Raton: CRC Press, Inc. pp. 39–58.

King JC, and Cousins RJ 2006. Zinc. *In*: Shils ME, Shike M, Ross AC, Caballero B, and Cousins RJ *Eds.* 2006. Modern Nutrition in Health and Disease. 10th ed. Baltimore: Lippincott Williams & Wilkins. pp. 271–285.

Kiremidjian-Schumacher L, Roy M, and Glickman R, *et al.* 2000. Selenium and immunocompetence in patients with head and neck cancer. *Biol. Trace Elem. Res.* 73(2): 97–111.

Kiremidjian-Schumacher L, Roy M, Wishe HI, Cohen MW, and Stotzky G 1994. Supplementation with selenium and human immune cell functions. II. Effect on cytotoxic lymphocytes and natural killer cells. *Biol. Trace Elem. Res.* 41(1–2): 115–127.

Klevay LM 2000. Cardiovascular disease from copper deficiency—a history. *J. Nutr.* 130(2S Suppl): 489S–492S.

Klipstein-Grobusch K, Grobbee DE, den Breeijen JH, Boeing H, Hofman A, and Witteman JC 1999. Dietary iron and risk of myocardial infarction in the Rotterdam Study. *Am. J. Epidemiol.* 149(5): 421–428.

Knekt P, Marniemi J, Teppo L, Heliovaara M, and Aromaa A 1998. Is low selenium status a risk factor for lung cancer? *Am. J. Epidemiol.* 148(10): 975–982.

Knochel JP, 2006. Phosphorus. *In*: Shils ME, Shike M, Ross AC, Caballero B, and Cousins RJ *Eds.* Modern Nutrition in Health and Disease. 10th ed. Baltimore: Lippincott Williams & Wilkins. pp. 211–222.

Kosar F, Sahin I, Acikgoz N, Aksoy Y, Kucukbay Z, and Cehreli S 2005. Significance of serum trace element status in patients with rheumatic heart disease: a prospective study. *Biol. Trace Elem. Res.* 107(1): 1–10.

Kupka R, and Fawzi W 2002. Zinc nutrition and HIV infection. *Nutr. Rev.* 60(3): 69–79.

Lai H, Lai S, Shor-Posner G, Ma F, Trapido E, and Baum MK 2001. Plasma zinc, copper, copper: zinc ratio, and survival in a cohort of HIV-1-infected homosexual men. *J. Acquir Immune Defic Syndr.* 27(1): 56–62.

Lalioti V, Muruais G, Tsuchiya Y, Pulido D, and Sandoval IV 2009. Molecular mechanisms of copper homeostasis. *Front Biosci.* 14: 4878–903.

Lawson KA, Wright ME, Subar A, *et al.* 2007. Multivitamin use and risk of prostate cancer in the National Institutes of Health-AARP Diet and Health Study. *J. Natl. Cancer Inst.* 99(10): 754–764.

Leone N, Courbon D, Ducimetiere P, and Zureik M 2006. Zinc, copper, and magnesium and risks for all-cause, cancer, and cardiovascular mortality. *Epidemiology* 17(3): 308–314.

Linder MC, and Hazegh-Azam M 1996. Copper biochemistry and molecular biology. *Am. J. Clin. Nutr.* 63(5): 797S–811S.

Lippman SM, Klein EA, Goodman PJ, *et al.* 2009. Effect of selenium and vitamin E on risk of prostate cancer and other cancers: the Selenium and Vitamin E Cancer Prevention Trial (SELECT). *JAMA* 301(1): 39–51.

Lobo JC, Torres JP, Fouque D, and Mafra D 2009. Zinc deficiency in chronic kidney disease: Is there a relationship with adipose tissue and atherosclerosis? *Biol. Trace Elem. Res.* [Epub ahead of print].

Luca E, Crivoi F, Gale C, Popescu E, Ciubotariu D, and Nechifor M 2009. Research on serum and saliva concentration of some bivalent cations in patient with suppurations of the oro-maxillo-facial area. *Rev. Med. Chir. Soc. Med. Nat. Iasi.* 113(3): 899–903.

Lukaski HC, 1999. Chromium as a supplement. *Annu Rev. Nutr.* 19: 279–302.

Lynch SR, 1997. Interaction of iron with other nutrients. *Nutr. Rev.* 55(4): 102–110.

MacDonald RS, 2000. The role of zinc in growth and cell proliferation. *J. Nutr.* 130(5S Suppl): 1500S–1508S.

Mahomed K, Bhutta Z, and Middleton P 2007. Zinc supplementation for improving pregnancy and infant outcome. *Cochrane Database Syst Rev.* 2: CD000230.

Malek F, Jiresova E, Dohnalova A, Koprivova H, and Spacek R 2006. Serum copper as a marker of inflammation in prediction of short term outcome in high risk patients with chronic heart failure. *Int. J. Cardiol.* 113(2): 51–53.

Mazariegos M, Hambidge KM, Westcott JE, Solomons NW, Raboy V, Das A, Goco N, Kindem M, Wright LL, and Krebs NF 2010. Neither a zinc supplement nor phytate-reduced maize nor their combination enhance growth of 6- to 12-Month-old guatemalan infants. *J. Nutr.* [Epub ahead of print].

Micronutrients: Linus Pauling Institute Micronutrient information center Oregon State University.

Mocchegiani E, and Muzzioli M 2000. Therapeutic application of zinc in human immunodeficiency virus against opportunistic infections. *J. Nutr.* 130(5S Suppl): 1424S–1431S.

Muller O, Becher H, van Zweeden AB, *et al.* 2001. Effect of zinc supplementation on malaria and other causes of morbidity in West African children: randomised double blind placebo controlled trial. *BMJ.* 322(7302): 1567.

Nomura AM, Lee J, Stemmermann GN, and Combs GF Jr 2000. Serum selenium and subsequent risk of prostate cancer. *Cancer Epidemiol Biomarkers Prev.* 9(9): 883–887.

O'Dell BL, 2000. Role of zinc in plasma membrane function. *J. Nutr*. 130(5S Suppl): 1432S–1436S.

Osendarp SJ, van Raaij JM, Arifeen SE, Wahed M, Baqui AH, and Fuchs GJ 2000. A randomized, placebo-controlled trial of the effect of zinc supplementation during pregnancy on pregnancy outcome in Bangladeshi urban poor. *Am. J. Clin. Nutr.* 71(1): 114–119.

Percival SS, Kauwell OP, Bowser E, and Wagner M 1999. Altered copper status in adult men with cystic fibrosis. *J. Am. Coll. Nutr.* 18(6): 614-619.

Peterson LN, 1997. Potassium in nutrition. *In*: O'Dell BL, and Sunde RA, *Eds*. Handbook of nutritionally essential minerals. New York: Marcel Dekker, Inc. pp. 153–183.

Pietrangelo A, 1998. Hemochromatosis is one gene enough? *J. Hepatol*. 29(3): 502–509.

Pinero DJ, Hu J, and Connor JR 2000. Alterations in the interaction between iron regulatory proteins and their iron responsive element in normal and Alzheimer's diseased brains. *Cell. Mol. Biol.* (Noisy-le-grand). 46(4): 761–776.

Prasad AS, 2009. Zinc: role in immunity, oxidative stress and chronic inflammation. *Curr. Opin. Clin. Nutr. Metab. Care*. 12(6): 646–52.

Prasad AS, Beck FW, Snell DC, and Kucuk O 2009. Zinc in cancer prevention. *Nutr. Cancer.* 61(6): 879–87.

Prasad AS, Fitzgerald JT, Bao B, Beck FW, and Chandrasekar PH 2000. Duration of symptoms and plasma cytokine levels in patients with the common cold treated with zinc acetate. A randomized, double-blind, placebo-controlled trial. *Ann. Intern. Med.* 133(4): 245–252.

Prasad AS, Halsted JA, and Nadimi M 1961. Syndrome of iron deficiency anemia, hepatosplenomegaly, hypogonadism, dwarfism, and geophagia. *Am. J. Med*. 31: 532–546.

Rajpathak S, Rimm E, Morris JS, and Hu F 2005. Toenail selenium and cardiovascular disease in men with diabetes. *J. Am. Coll. Nutr*. 24(4): 250–256.

Rayman MP, 2000. The importance of selenium to human health. *Lancet*. 356(9225): 233–241.

Rivera-Mancía S, Pérez-Neri I, Ríos C, Tristán-López L, Rivera-Espinosa L, and Montes S 2010. The transition metals copper and iron in neurodegenerative diseases. *Chem. Biol. Interact*. 186(2): 184–99.

Roels H, Lauwerys R, Buchet JP, *et al.* 1987. Epidemiological survey among workers exposed to manganese: effects on lung, central nervous system, and some biological indices. *Am. J. Ind. Med*. 11(3): 307–327.

Roozbeh J, Hedayati P, Sagheb MM, Sharifian M, Jahromi AH, Shaabani S, Jalaeian H, Raeisjalali GA, and Behzadi S 2009. Effect of zinc supplementation on triglyceride, cholesterol, LDL, and HDL levels in zinc-deficient hemodialysis patients. *Ren. Fail*. 31(9): 798–801.

Roy M, Kiremidjian-Schumacher L, Wishe HI, Cohen MW, and Stotzky G 1994. Supplementation with selenium and human immune cell functions. I. Effect on lymphocyte proliferation and interleukin 2 receptor expression. *Biol. Trace Elem. Res*. 41(1–2): 103–114.

Saaka M, Oosthuizen J, and Beatty S 2009. Effect of joint iron and zinc supplementation on malarial infection and anaemia. *East Afr. J. Public Health*. 6(1): 55–62.

Saaka M, Oosthuizen J, and Beatty S 2009. Effect of prenatal zinc supplementation on birthweight. *J. Health Popul. Nutr*. 27(5): 619–31.

Sachdev H, Gera T, and Nestel P 2005. Effect of iron supplementation on mental and motor development in children: systematic review of randomised controlled trials. *Public Health Nutr*. 8(2): 117–132.

Salgueiro MJ, Zubillaga M, Lysionek A, *et al.* 2000. Zinc status and immune system relationship: a review. *Biol. Trace Elem. Res.* 76(3): 193–205.

Salonen JT, Alfthan G, Huttunen JK, Pikkarainen J, and Puska P 1982. Association between cardiovascular death and myocardial infarction and serum selenium in a matched-pair longitudinal study. *Lancet*. 2(8291): 175–179.

Salvador GA. Iron in neuronal function and dysfunction. *Biofactors*. 36(2): 103–10.

Salvini S, Hennekens CH, Morris JS, Willett WC, and Stampfer MJ 1995. Plasma levels of the antioxidant selenium and risk of myocardial infarction among U.S. physicians. *Am. J. Cardiol*. 76(17): 1218–1221.

Sánchez C, López-Jurado M, Aranda P, and Llopis J 2010. Plasma levels of copper, manganese and selenium in an adult population in southern Spain: influence of age, obesity and lifestyle factors. *Sci. Total Environ*. 408(5): 1014–20.

Saper RB, and Rash R 2009. Zinc: an essential micronutrient. *Am Fam Physician*. 79(9): 768–72.

Sayre LM, Perry G, Atwood CS, and Smith MA 2000. The role of metals in neurodegenerative diseases. *Cell. Mol. Biol*. 46(4): 731–741.

Sazawal S, Black RE, Ramsan M, *et al.* 2007. Effect of zinc supplementation on mortality in children aged 1-48 months: a community-based randomised placebo-controlled trial. *Lancet*. 369(9565): 927–934.

Shah D, and Sachdev HP 2006. Zinc deficiency in pregnancy and fetal outcome. *Nutr. Rev*. 64(1): 15–30.

Shankar AH, 2000. Nutritional modulation of malaria morbidity and mortality. *J. Infect Dis.* 182(Suppl 1): S37–53.

Shils ME, 1997. Magnesium. *In*: O'Dell BL, and Sunde RA, *Eds*. Handbook of nutritionally essential minerals. New York: Marcel Dekker, Inc. pp. 117–152.

Smith W, Mitchell P, Webb K, and Leeder SR, 1999. Dietary antioxidants and age-related maculopathy: the Blue Mountains Eye Study. *Ophthalmology*. 106(4): 761–767.

Song Y, Elias V, Loban A, Scrimgeour AG, and Ho E 2010. Marginal zinc deficiency increases oxidative DNA damage in the prostate after chronic exercise. *Free Radic Biol. Med.* 48(1): 82–8.

Spencer H, Norris C, and Williams D 1994. Inhibitory effects of zinc on magnesium balance and magnesium absorption in man. *J. Am. Coll. Nutr*. 13(5): 479–484.

Stern BR 2010. Essentiality and toxicity in copper health risk assessment: overview, update and regulatory considerations. *J. Toxicol. Environ. Health A*. 73(2): 114–27.

Stoecker BJ, 1999. Chromium. *In*: Shils M, Olson JA, Shike M, and Ross AC *Eds*. Nutrition in Health and Disease. 9th ed. Baltimore: Williams & Wilkins. pp. 277–282.

Stranges S, Marshall JR, Natarajan R, *et al.* 2007. Effects of long-term selenium supplementation on the incidence of type 2 diabetes: A randomized trial. *Ann. Intern. Med.* 147(4): 217–223.

Suadicani P, Hein HO, and Gyntelberg F 1992. Serum selenium concentration and risk of ischaemic heart disease in a prospective cohort study of 3000 males. *Atherosclerosis* 96(1): 33–42.

Suharno D, West CE, Muhilal, Karyadi D, and Hautvast JG 1993. Supplementation with vitamin A and iron for nutritional anaemia in pregnant women in West Java, Indonesia. *Lancet*. 342(8883): 1325–1328

Szajewska H, Ruszczynski M, and Chmielewska A 2010. Effects of iron supplementation in nonanemic pregnant women, infants, and young children on the mental performance and psychomotor development of children: a systematic review of randomized controlled trials. *Am. J. Clin. Nutr.* 91(6): 1684–90.

Szewczyk B, Kubera M, and Nowak G 2010. The role of zinc in neurodegenerative inflammatory pathways in depression. *Prog. Neuropsychopharmacol Biol. Psychiatry*. [Epub ahead of print].

Takaoka T, Sarukura N, Ueda C, *et al.* 2010. Effects of zinc supplementation on serum zinc concentration and ratio of apo/holo-activities of angiotensin converting enzyme in patients with taste impairment. *Auris Nasus Larynx*. 37(2): 190–4.

Taubes G 1998. The (political) science of salt. *Science*. 281(5379): 898–901, 903–897.

The United Nations Children's Fund/World Health Organization. WHO/UNICEF Joint Statement: Clinical Management of Acute Diarrhoea. Geneva; New York; 2004:1-8. Available at: http://www.unicef.org/publications/index_21433.html.

The Zinc Against Plasmodium Study Group effect of zinc on the treatment of *Plasmodium falciparum* malaria in children: a randomized controlled trial. *Am. J. Clin. Nutr*. 2002; 76(4): 805–812.

Thomas DG, Grant SL, and Aubuchon-Endsley NL 2009. The role of iron in neurocognitive development. *Dev. Neuropsychol*. 34(2): 196–222.

Thompson CA, Habermann TM, Wang AH, Vierkant RA, Folsom AR, Ross JA, and Cerhan JR 2010. Antioxidant intake from fruits, vegetables and other sources and risk of non-Hodgkin's lymphoma: the Iowa Women's Health Study. *Int J. Cancer*. 126(4): 992–1003.

Truong-Tran AQ, Ho LH, Chai F, and Zalewski PD 2000. Cellular zinc fluxes and the regulation of apoptosis/gene-directed cell death. *J. Nutr*. 130(5S Suppl): 1459S–1466S.

Tuerk MJ, and Fazel N 2009. Zinc deficiency. *Curr. Opin. Gastroenterol*. 25(2): 136–43.

Tupe R, and Agte V 2009. An *in vitro* study for antiglycation role of zinc along with ascorbic acid and folic acid in BSA glycation. *British J. Nutr*. 103: 370–377.

Tupe R, and Agte V 2010. Effect of water soluble vitamins on Zn transport of Caco-2 cells and their implications under oxidative stress conditions, available online with *European J. Nutr.* 49: 53–61.

Tupe R, Tupe S, Tarwadi K, and Agte V 2010. Effect of different dietary zinc levels on hepatic antioxidant and micronutrients indices under oxidative stress conditions' Metabolism. 59: 1603–1611.

Tupe RS, Chiplonkar SA, and Agte VV 2007. Changes in zinc uptake in response to ascorbic acid and folic acid in rat liver slices under normal and oxidative stress conditions *Bio. Factors* 30(1): 27–34.

Turner RB, and Cetnarowski WE 2000. Effect of treatment with zinc gluconate or zinc acetate on experimental and natural colds. *Clin. Infect Dis.* 31(5): 1202–1208.

Turnlund JR 2006. Copper. *In*: Shils ME, Shike M, Ross AC, Caballero B, and Cousins RJ, *Eds*. Modern Nutrition in Health and Disease. 10th ed. Philadelphia: Lippincott Williams & Wilkins. 286–299.

Uauy R, Olivares M, and Gonzalez M 1998. Essentiality of copper in humans. *Am J. Clin. Nutr.* 67(5 Suppl): 952S–959S.

Umusig-Quitain P, and Gregorio GV 2010. High incidence of zinc deficiency among Filipino children with compensated and decompensated liver disease. *J. Gastroenterol Hepatol.* 25(2): 387–90.

Van den Berghe PV, and Klomp LW 2009. New developments in the regulation of intestinal copper absorption. *Nutr. Rev.* 67(11): 658–72.

Van der AD, Peeters PH, Grobbee DE, Marx JJ, and van der Schouw YT 2005. Dietary haem iron and coronary heart disease in women. *Eur. Heart. J.* 26(3): 257–262.

VandenLangenberg GM, Mares-Perlman JA, Klein R, Klein BE, Brady WE, and Palta M 1998. Associations between antioxidant and zinc intake and the 5-year incidence of early age-related maculopathy in the Beaver Dam Eye Study. *Am. J. Epidemiol.* 148(2): 204–214.

Virtamo J, Valkeila E, Alfthan G, Punsar S, Huttunen JK, and Karvonen MJ 1985. Serum selenium and the risk of coronary heart disease and stroke. *Am J. Epidemiol.* 122(2): 276–282.

Vulpe CD, Kuo YM, Murphy TL, *et al.* 1999. Hephaestin, a ceruloplasmin homologue implicated in intestinal iron transport, is defective in the Sla mouse. *Nat. Genet.* 21(2): 195–199.

Walravens PA, Hambidge KM, and Koepfer DM 1989. Zinc supplementation in infants with a nutritional pattern of failure to thrive: a double-blind, controlled study. *Pediatrics.* 83(4): 532–538.

Wasserman GA, Liu X, Parvez F, *et al.* 2006. Water manganese exposure and children's intellectual function in Araihazar, Bangladesh. *Environ. Health Perspect.* 114(1): 124–129.

Weaver CM, and Heaney RP 1999. Calcium. *In*: Shils M, Olson JA, Shike M, and Ross AC, *Eds*. Modern Nutrition in Health and Disease. 9th ed. Baltimore: Williams & Wilkins. pp. 141–155.

Wellinghausen N, Kern WV, Jochle W, and Kern P 2000. Zinc serum level in human immunodeficiency virus-infected patients in relation to immunological status. *Biol. Trace Elem. Res.* 73(2): 139–149.

Whanger PD, 2004. Selenium and its relationship to cancer: an update. *Br J. Nutr.* 91(1): 11–28.

Wood RJ, and Ronnenberg AG 2006. Iron. *In*: Shils ME, Shike M, and Ross AC, Caballero B, and Cousins RJ, *Eds*. Modern Nutrition in Health and Disease. 10th ed. Philadelphia: Lippincott Williams & Wilkins. pp. 248–270.

World Cancer Research Fund/American Institute for Cancer Research 2007. Food, Nutrition, Physical Activity, and the Prevention of Cancer: a Global Perspective. Washington, D.C.: AICR.

Wright RO, Amarasiriwardena C, Woolf AD, Jim R, and Bellinger DC 2006. Neuropsychological correlates of hair arsenic, manganese, and cadmium levels in school-age children residing near a hazardous waste site. *Neurotoxicology* 27(2): 210–216.

Wuebbens MM, Liu MT, Rajagopalan K, and Schindelin H 2000. Insights into molybdenum cofactor deficiency provided by the crystal structure of the molybdenum cofactor biosynthesis protein MoaC. *Structure Fold Des.* 8(7): 709–718.

Wurzelmann JI, Silver A, Schreinemachers DM, Sandler RS, and Everson RB 1996. Iron intake and the risk of colorectal cancer. *Cancer Epidemiol Biomarkers Prev*. 5(7): 503–507.

Yamaguchi M, 2009. Role of nutritional zinc in the prevention of osteoporosis. *Mol. Cell Biochem*. 338(1-2): 241–254.

Yip R, 2000. Significance of an abnormally low or high hemoglobin concentration during pregnancy: special consideration of iron nutrition. *Am. J. Clin. Nutr.* 72(1 Suppl): 272S–279S.

Yip R, and Dallman PR 1996. Iron. *In*: Ziegler EE, and Filer LJ, *Eds*. Present Knowledge in Nutrition. 7th ed. Washington D.C.: ILSI Press. pp. 277–292.

Yoshizawa K, Willett WC, Morris SJ, *et al.* 1998. Study of prediagnostic selenium level in toenails and the risk of advanced prostate cancer. *J. Natl. Cancer Inst.* 90(16): 1219–1224.

Yu MW, Horng IS, Hsu KH, Chiang YC, Liaw YF, and Chen CJ 1999. Plasma selenium levels and risk of hepatocellular carcinoma among men with chronic hepatitis virus infection. *Am. J. Epidemiol.* 150(4): 367–374.

Zhang W, Ramanathan CS, Nadimpalli RG, Bhat AA, Cox AG, and Taylor EW 1999. Selenium-dependent glutathione peroxidase modules encoded by RNA viruses. *Biol. Trace Elem. Res.* 70(2): 97–116.

Zhao L, Cox AG, Ruzicka JA, Bhat AA, Zhang W, and Taylor EW 2000. Molecular modeling and *in vitro* activity of an HIV-1-encoded glutathione peroxidase. *Proc. Natl. Acad. Sci. USA* 97(12): 6356–6361.

Zhong W, McClain CJ, Cave M, Kang YJ, and Zhou Z 2010. The role of zinc deficiency in alcohol-induced intestinal barrier dysfunction. *Am J. Physiol Gastrointest Liver Physiol.* 298(5): 6625–33.

Zhuo H, Smith AH, and Steinmaus C 2004. Selenium and lung cancer: a quantitative analysis of heterogeneity in the current epidemiological literature. *Cancer Epidemiol Biomarkers Prev.* 13(5): 771–778.

4

Antioxidants: The Biological Fire Fighters

Oxidation is a crucial reaction required for sustaining life, but it can also turn out to be harmful when excess free radicals are produced, which start chain reactions that damage cells. Free radicals are unstable molecules that essentially steal away electrons from otherwise healthy molecules in order to survive. Every day, several free radicals get generated within the body, causing a risk of cell damage that can lead to chronic and degenerative diseases if left uncontrolled. Such molecules come in the form of synthetic chemicals such as pesticides, plastics, and chlorine byproducts and are called precursors of free radicals. Antioxidants are the natural molecules having capacity to quench these potentially dangerous reactive molecules in the body.

It is ironic that oxygen, an element indispensable for life, under certain situations, has severely deleterious effects on the human body. Reactive oxygen species (ROS) is a collective term that implies to oxygen radicals and certain non-radicals, which are oxidizing agents and/or are easily converted into radicals. The oxygen containing free radicals include superoxide (O_2.-),hydroxyl (OH.), peroxyl (RO_2.), alkoxyl (RO.) and hydroperoxyl (HO_2.), while hydrogen peroxide (H_2O_2), hypochlorus acid (HOCl), ozone (O_3) and singlet oxygen (O_2.) are among the non radicals. Generation of these radicals can result into oxidative stress.

An antioxidant can be defined as a molecule capable of slowing or preventing the oxidation of other molecules. Both, plants and animals maintain complex systems of multiple types of antioxidants, such as glutathione, vitamin C, and vitamin E as well as enzymes such as catalase, superoxide dismutase and various peroxidases. Low levels of antioxidants, or inhibition of the antioxidant enzymes, in presence of excess free radicals, cause oxidative stress and may have detrimental effects on cells. Antioxidants terminate the chain reactions by removing free radical intermediates, and inhibit other oxidation reactions by getting oxidized themselves. As a result, antioxidants are often reducing agents such as thiols, ascorbic acid or polyphenols (Sies, 1997).

The body can sometimes create its own free radicals in order to destroy viruses or bacteria. To balance out these uncontrollable molecules, the body also creates antioxidants, which have the only purpose of neutralizing free radicals. However, human body can create only certain amount of antioxidants on its own and when it faces large number of environmental toxins, the body is unable to handle the load of these unwanted molecules. Fruits and vegetables provide the body with an added source of antioxidants needed to properly fight against free radicals. Without the necessary intake of healthy fruits and vegetables, free radicals can spread and eventually lead to stroke, heart attack, arthritis, vision problems, Parkinson's disease, Alzheimer's disease and various types of cancer. The benefits of having sufficient daily intake of fruits and vegetables are enormous.

Fruit and vegetables are a major source of antioxidants, particularly vitamins C and E and the carotenoids. This explains why diets rich in these foods appear to have a protective effect against cancer and heart disease and many other disorders including infertility etc. Among the factors that influence cellular response and susceptibility to environmental agents, diet has received increased attention in recent years. While the modes of action are complex and multifarious, increased oxidative stress is directly or indirectly responsible for causing and or aggravating the adverse effects from exposure to a number of environmental agents (Cookson, 1999).

The antioxidant, vitamin E, is considered good for the heart since it has the ability to essentially reduce the LDL cholesterol in our arteries, allowing for the necessary elasticity and blood pressure levels to keep our heart pumping safely. Cholesterol, if left untreated, builds up as plaque on the inside walls of the arteries, impeding blood flow of LDL and forcing the heart to overwork. If the built up plaque is severe, it can create a blockage in the artery, leading to heart attack or stroke. By getting enough vitamin E through diet, one can protect body through other necessary antioxidants to prevent LDL cholesterol levels to rise.

Antioxidants can protect against diabetes related oxidative damage. Free radicals increase in the altered metabolic states of diabetics. But with the sufficient antioxidants that fruits and vegetables can provide, free radicals can be quenched, protecting the kidneys, blood vessels, eyes and heart from harmful damage. Free radicals support cancer cells growth. Many studies have linked cancer of the stomach, prostate, colon, breast, bladder, esophagus and pancreas, to free radicals. Eating fruits and vegetables may not prevent cancer, but can give our body the fighting molecules that it needs.

Antioxidants also have been shown to slow down the effects of aging. Free radicals damage the cells within our body that are needed to a youthful appearance and good health. Eating fruits and vegetables can slow down the loss of muscle elasticity which leads to wrinkles, boost the immunity making our body less susceptible to illness, and also put the breaks on memory failure, as free radicals injure the brain cells that are necessary for retaining information.

Antioxidants are available in supplement form but are more powerful when found in whole foods. Leafy vegetables and orange colored fruits and vegetables are excellent sources of the antioxidant beta-carotene. Fruits and vegetables containing lycopene, such as tomatoes, watermelon, guava, papaya, apricots and pink grapefruit, are also rich in antioxidants. But it is important that fruits and vegetables are grown using organic farming so that these will be free from pesticides. Eating of fruits and vegetables with non-organic practices may not give the desirable amounts of antioxidants (or vitamins and minerals) that our body needs. On average, organic produce contains nearly 30% more nutrients than non-organic and is grown without using harsh chemicals that can lead to further free radical exposure.

The research during last decade has clearly indicated oxidative stress to be an important etiological factor of many human diseases. Consequently, organisms contain a complex network of antioxidant metabolites and enzymes that work together to prevent oxidative damage to cellular components such as DNA, proteins and lipids (Sies 1997, Vertuani *et al.,* 2004). Antioxidants have been suggested as the adjunct therapy in many non communicable diseases, particularly for stroke and neurodegenerative diseases. Antioxidants are also widely used as ingredients in dietary supplements in management and prevention of cancer and coronary heart disease. But, large clinical trials have not been conclusive about the benefit and have suggested some caution about excess supplementation of antioxidants which may be harmful (Bjelakovic *et al.,* 2007). In general, antioxidant systems either prevent these reactive species from being formed, or remove them before they can damage vital components of the cell (Sies, 1997; Davies, 1995). However, since reactive oxygen species do have some useful functions in cells, like redox signaling, the function of antioxidant systems is not to remove oxidants entirely, but instead to keep them at an optimum level (Rhee, June 2006).

Enzymatic pathway for detoxification of reactive oxygen species

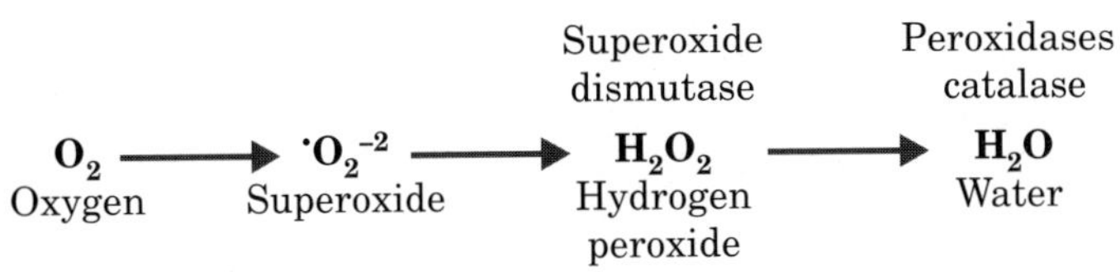

As with the chemical antioxidants, cells are protected against oxidative stress by an interacting network of antioxidant enzymes (Sies 1997; Davies, 1995). The superoxide released by processes such as oxidative phosphorylation is first converted to hydrogen peroxide and then further reduced to give water. This detoxification pathway is the result of multiple enzymes, with superoxide dismutases catalysing the first step followed by catalases and various peroxidases removing hydrogen peroxide.

Superoxide dismutases (SODs) are referred as group of closely related enzymes that catalyze the breakdown of the superoxide anion into oxygen and hydrogen peroxide (Zelko *et al.,* 2002; Bannister *et al.,* 1987). SODs are present in almost all aerobic cells and in extracellular fluids (Johnson and Giulivi, 2005). Superoxide dismutase enzymes contain metal ion as cofactors which, depending on the isozyme, can be copper, zinc, manganese or iron. In humans, the copper/zinc SOD is present in the cytosol, while manganese SOD is present in the mitochondrion (Bannister *et al.,* 1987). There is also a third form of SOD in extracellular fluids, which contains copper and zinc in its active sites (Nozik-Grayck *et al.,* 2005). Catalases are enzymes which catalyse the conversion of hydrogen peroxide to water and oxygen, using either an iron or manganese as their cofactor (Chelikani *et al.,* 2004; Zámocký and Koller, 1999).

OXIDATIVE STRESS AND ANTIOXIDANTS

Oxidative stress is a term used to describe any challenge in which pro-oxidants predominate over antioxidants; it may be due to either increased production of ROS or decreased levels of antioxidants (enzymatic and nonenzymatic) or both. Oxidative stress is a major contributing factor in certain disorders such as diabetes, cataract, cancer and cardiovascular disorder (CVD).

Oxidative stress has been an aetiological factor in the development of Alzheimer's disease, Parkinson's disease (Christen Y, 2000; Nunomura *et al.,* 2006; Wood-Kaczmar *et al.,* 2006), the pathologies caused by diabetes rheumatoid arthritis (Davi, 2006; Giugliano *et al.,* 1996; Hitchon and El-Gabalawy, 2004) and neurodegeneration in motor neuron diseases (Cookson and Shaw, 1999). In these diseases, it is unclear if oxidants trigger the disease, or if they are produced as a secondary consequence of the disease and from general tissue damage; One case in which this link is particularly well-understood is the role of oxidative stress in cardiovascular disease wherin low density lipoprotein (LDL) oxidation appears to trigger the process of atherogenesis, which results in atherosclerosis, and finally cardiovascular disease (Van Gaal *et al.,* 2006, Aviram, 2000).

Antioxidants are broadly classified into two divisions, depending on whether they are soluble in water (hydrophilic) or in lipids (hydrophobic). In general, water-soluble antioxidants react with oxidants present in the cell cytosol and the blood plasma, while lipid-soluble antioxidants protect mainly the cell membranes from lipid peroxidation (Sies, 1997). These compounds may be synthesized in the body or obtained from the diet (Vertuani *et al.,* 2004). Some compounds function in antioxidant defense by chelating transition metals and preventing these metals from catalyzing the production of free radicals in the cell. Particularly important is the ability of these compounds to sequester iron, which is the function of iron-binding proteins such as transferrin and ferritin (Imlay, 2003). Selenium and zinc are commonly referred to as 'antioxidant micronutrients', but these do not have antioxidant action by themselves and are instead required for the activity of some antioxidant enzymes.

***Polyphenols*:** Polyphenols are types of antioxidants containing a polyphenolic substructure. There are over 4,000 such distinct compounds that have antioxidant activity *in vitro* but their antioxidant roles *in vivo* are not yet confirmed (Williams *et al.,* 2004; Frei, 2009). The main sources of polyphenols in foods are fruits like apples, blackberries, cherries, grapes, pears, plums, raspberries, and strawberries; and vegetables like cabbage, celery, onion. Red wine, honey, chocolate, green tea, olive oil, bee pollen and grains like sorghum are also the sources. Various reactive oxygen species, such as singlet oxygen, peroxynitrite and hydrogen peroxide, must be continually removed from cells to maintain healthy metabolic function. The mechanism of a polyphenol antioxidant's ability is by scavenging free radicals and to up-regulate certain metal chelation reactions.

Beneficial effects of dietary polyphenols

- Improved endothelial function via down regulation of oxidative LDL (Serafini *et al.*, 2000).
- Anti-inflammatory effects as seen in coronary artery disease (Muldoon *et al.*, 1996; Zimmer *et al.*, 2002).
- Reducing reactive oxygen species levels *in vitro* as shown by tea polyphenol antioxidant epigallocatechin gallate (EGCG) (Mei *et al.*, 2005).
- Inhibiting occurrence and/or growth of experimental tumors exhibited by some polyphenols, like resveratrol (Jang *et al.*, 1997).
- Anti-aging effects such as slowing the process of skin wrinkling (Vieira *et al.*, 1998).

It is difficult to separate the physiological effects of individual polyphenol, since there are large number of such compounds which may occur even in a single food and their fate *in vivo* is difficult to be measured. For example, over sixty different chemically distinct flavonoids are known to occur in a given red wine and has a high polyphenol content of up to 2-3 grams per litre. Other reports have also elucidated the difficulty of isolating individual polyphenolic antioxidants. Moreover, significant biodiversity occurs in polyphenol content among various foods leading to inconsistencies of epidemiological studies implying beneficial health effects of polyphenol antioxidants (Lirai *et al.,* 2002).

There is debate about absorption of dietary polyphenols. While some studies do indicate potential health effects of certain specific polyphenols, most studies also have demonstrated low bioavailability and rapid excretion of polyphenols, limiting their potential roles *in vivo* being in small concentrations (Williams *et al.,* 2004; Frei 2009; Virgili and Marino, 2008). More research is needed to understand the interactions between polyphenols present as combinations within the human body. There are reports that some foods may actually inhibit bioavailability of polyphenols such as refined sugars, which have shown to impede the uptake under certain circumstances. Furthermore, caution should be exercised in trying diets depending largely on dietary supplements as opposed to a broad array of food sources, since the quality and levels of useful molecules in some commercial products may be questionable.

***Phytates and phytic acid*:** Phytates are phosphate esters of inositol found primarily in cereal grains, legumes, and nuts. They bind with minerals such as iron, calcium, and zinc and inhibit their absorption in the body. Phytic acid present in cereals, legumes and oilseeds was earlier regarded as an anti-nutritive factor. It's inhibitory effects on the bioavailabilty of iron and other essential minerals and trace elements have been described in several studies in man and monogastric animals. Phytic acid and iron are considered to form insoluble complexes due to which these are are not available for absorption under the pH conditions of the small intestine. A number of recent studies have suggested that reducing the phytate content of foods by genetic modification or by the action of intrinsic or extrinsic phytases can have a beneficial effect on iron availability. Over the last decade potential beneficial effects of phytic acid have also been recognized. For expample, *in vitro* studies indicate that phytic acid acts as an anti-oxidant through its iron chelating properties. However, it is as yet uncertain whether physiological intakes of phytic acid can significantly improve the anti-oxidant status in man and animals (Minihane *et al.,* 2002).

Phytates/phytic acid are the storage forms of phosphorus in the bran fiber of raw whole grains. Even if some foods have a high phosphorus content, the phosphates in phytates are not released through the digestive process due to lack of phytases. When bread is leavened by yeast, lactic acid bacteria or natural flora, the phytases get activated hydrolyzing the phytates and increasing the trace metal bioavailability (Agte *et al.,* 1997). Phytic acid is also destroyed during baking and sprouting of seeds, grains, legumes, the roasting of nuts, presoaking beans, cooking, fermentation, combining acidic foods with zinc-rich foods and food processing such as soaking the batter (Agte and Joshi, 1997; Agte *et al.,* 1998 and 1999).

Current understanding of phytates no more considers them to be antinutritional factors. Although phytates bind with minerals, this ability may actually be preventing the formation of free radicals, thereby keeping the minerals at safe levels in the body. In this sense phytates act as antioxidants. Some animal studies have suggested that phytates stop the growth of cancerous tumors.

Scientists are beginning to express concern over excess iron in the body due to its prooxidant effect in reduced form Fe^{2+}. Excessive iron is also known to increase the risk of heart disease. Even a small amount of phytates in food can reduce iron absorption by half, but the effect is less severe if a meal is supplemented with ascorbic acid, which can also help the absorption of zinc and calcium. Phytates are generally found in foods high in fiber. Since fiber-rich foods protect against colon and breast cancers, it is now thought that they are the protective agent in the fiber. By binding minerals in the intestines, phytates inhibit the cancer process, especially when it comes to iron which generates free radicals.

Phytates are also known to help prevent cancer by enhancing the immune system. Phytates may increase the activity of natural killer cells which attack and destroy cancer cells and tumors. By working directly to control cell growth, phytates may be an ideal protective agent against a wide range of cancers, carrying excess minerals out of the body, thereby protecting it from a potential overload. Fiber, along with its associated phytates, also provides benefits by regulating the absorption of glucose from starch.

The catalysis by iron of radical formation and subsequent oxidative damage has been well documented. Although many iron-chelating agents potentiate reactive oxygen formation and lipid peroxidation, phytic acid which is abundant in edible legumes, cereals, and seeds forms an iron chelate which greatly accelerates Fe^{2+}-mediated oxygen reduction yet blocks iron-driven hydroxyl radical generation and suppresses lipid peroxidation. Furthermore, high concentrations of phytic acid prevent browning and putrefaction of various fruits and vegetables by inhibiting polyphenol oxidase. These observations indicate an important antioxidant function for phytate in seeds during dormancy and suggest that phytate may be a substitute for presently employed preservatives, many of which pose potential health hazards (Graf *et al.,* 1987).

ANTIOXIDANT DEFENSE SYSTEM

The intracellular defense system largely depends on antioxidant enzymes, which are, glutathione peroxidase (GSH-PO), superoxide dismutase (SOD) and catalase (CAT) that require the antioxidant microelements. Selenium (Se) is chief constituent of GSH-PO, an enzyme important in the decomposition of hydrogen peroxide and lipid peroxides. Copper (Cu) is constituent of cytosolic SOD, which quenches the super oxide anions, and is also an ingredient for ceruloplasmin. Zinc (Zn) is also a chief constituent of cytosolic SOD; Manganese (Mn) is major component of mitochondrial SOD, whereas for CAT, a hemeprotein, that catalyzes the decomposition of H_2O_2, iron (Fe) is required for effective functioning. Riboflavin functions as an antioxidant since it is needed as a co-factor as Flavin Adenine Dinucleotide (FAD) for glutathione reductase (GSH-R) (Duncan, 1981).

FREE RADICALS AND ANTIOXIDANTS

Free radicals are chemical species with one or more unpaired electrons in their outer orbital. Our body normally produces them as they are normal byproducts of metabolism. However, uncontrolled generation of free radicals is destructive to the cells, tissues and organs. An understanding of free radical production due to external and internal sources and the intra- and extra- cellular defense mechanism which protect the cells against free radical toxicity is desirable in the face of continuous environmental disorders. Currently, most diseases including environmental disorders are linked with free radicals and their suppressors, the antioxidants (Slater, 1982; Tolonen, 1990).

Antioxidants not only support vital organs and systems through the detoxification process, but also curtail free radical activity. Free radicals damage underlies most degenerative diseases and heavy metal toxins have the ability to increase the production of free radicals within the body substantially (Ercal *et al.*, 2001). Indeed most of the damage caused by heavy metals stems from the oxidative free radicals. With a heavy toxic load, or antioxidant deficiencies, uncontrolled free radical production occurs. Antioxidants are defined as substances that when present at a much lower concentration than oxidisable substrate may significantly retard or prevent its oxidation.

Antioxidants play crucial roles in mammals and plants in protection against the harmful effects of free radicals generated during aerobic metabolism or through the action on xenobiotics (Arias and Jakoby, 1976; Foyer, 1994). By efficiently scavenging these free radicals, they prevent damage to DNA and lipids. Maintenance of the body's abundance of antioxidant concentrations such as vitamin A, C, E and β-carotene (all derivable from agricultural produce – fruits and vegetables). The molecular structure of these compounds is such that they can readily transfer a hydrogen atom to reactive free radicals, thus eliminating their deleterious effects. The resultant unpaired electron on the derivative of the antioxidant is so delocalized that it is also relatively innocuous.

Additionally, antioxidants break the vicious circle which involves the decomposition of fatty acids and proteins, the creation of new free radicals and eventual cell death. Selenium, zinc, manganese, ubiquinone (Q_{10}), vitamins A, C, E and some of the B vitamins, α-carotene, canthaxanthine, amino acids and other substances like certain drugs are effective antioxidants.

Fruits and vegetables are rich in vitamins which act as antioxidants. (RRI, 1995). There is a growing awareness that the occurence of certain diseases, including cancer and coronary heart disease is related to diet. (Ames 1983; McBrien and Slater 1992). The damage to DNA and lipids which precipitates the diseases can be induced by free radicals which in turn can be induced by environmental pollution (Shakman, 1974; Medeiros *et al.*, 1983). These radicals are normally scavenged and rendered unreactive by cellular antioxidants, many of which are vitamins or enzymes with trace elements as cofactors.

The brain due to its high metabolic rate and increased levels of polyunsaturated lipids is the target of lipid peroxidation and consequent oxidative injury (Aggarwal and Shishodia, 2006). Since fruits and vegetables happen to be good sources of antioxidants, they might prevent some types of diseases. Antioxidants from fruits and vegetables are also investigated as possible treatments for Alzheimer's disease, Parkinson's disease, heart disease and cancer (Kopke *et al.,* 2007; Stanner *et al.,* 2004). However, isolated antioxidant supplements have not shown clear effect on the risk of chronic diseases such as cancer and heart disease (Kopke *et al.,* 2007). This suggests that these health benefits be due to other substances in fruits and vegetables or from a complex mix of substances.

Oxidation of low density lipoprotein in the blood has been related to heart disease and initial observational studies taking vitamin E supplements had been found to have lower risk of developing heart disease (Lotito and Frei, 2006). Later large clinical trials were conducted to test the effects of vitamin E as supplement as 50 to 600 mg per day. None of these trials found a statistically significant effect of vitamin E on overall number of deaths or on deaths due to heart disease. While several trials have investigated supplements with high doses of antioxidants, the study by Cook *et al.* (2007) assessed the effect of supplementation with doses comparable to those in a healthy diet. Over 12,500 French men and women took either low-dose antioxidants (120 mg of ascorbic acid, 30 mg of vitamin E, 6 mg of beta carotene, 100 μg of selenium, and 20 mg of zinc) or placebo pills for an average of 7.5 years. The investigators found that there was no statistically significant effect of the antioxidants on overall survival, cancer, or heart disease. In a post-hoc analysis they found a 31% reduction in the risk of cancer in men, but not women.

In nutshell, antioxidants are the key molecules which keep the delicate balance of reactive oxygen species and prevent the damage due to their exposure manifested in many NCDS.

The principal message is that individuals and populations can protect themselves from decomposition and the ravages of environmental disorders by ensuring that they receive sufficient antioxidants.

REFERENCES

Aggarwal B, and Shishodia S 2006. Molecular targets of dietary agents for prevention and therapy of cancer. *Biochem. Pharmacol.* 71(10): 1397–421.

Agte V, and Joshi S 1997. Effect of traditional processing on phytate degradation in wheat and millets. *J. Agri. Food Chem.* 45: 1659–1661.

Agte V, Gokhale M, and Chiplonkar S 1997. Effects of fermentation on zinc bioavailability. *Int. J. Food. Sc. and Tech.*, 32: 29–32.

Agte V, Gokhale M, and Paknikar K 1999. Strategies for improving bioavailable amounts of iron and zinc from vegetarian meals: yeast fermentation and addition of legumes. *J. Food Sc. Tech.* 36: 551–554.

Agte V, Khot S, Joshi S, Chiplonkar S, and Paknikar K 1998. Effect of traditional processing of legumes on trace metal bioavailability. *J. Food Sc. Tech* 35: 330–332.

Ames B, 1983. Dietary carcinogens and anticarcinogens. Oxygen radicals and degenerative diseases. *Science* 221: 1256–63.

Arias B, and Jacoby W 1976. Role of reduced glutathione in delta-3-ketosteroid isomerase reaction. *Biochem. Biophys Res. Commu.* 69(4): 1073–79.

Aviram M, 2000. Review of human studies on oxidative damage and antioxidant protection related to cardiovascular diseases. *Free Radic. Res.* 33Suppl: S85–97.

Bannister J, Bannister W, and Rotilio G 1987. Aspects of the structure, function, and applications of superoxide dismutase. *CRC Crit Rev Biochem* 22(2): 111–80.

Bjelakovic G, Nikolova, D, Gluud, L, Simonetti R, and Gluud, C 2007. Mortality in randomized trials of antioxidant supplements for primary and secondary prevention: systematic review and meta-analysis. *JAMA* 297(8): 842–57.

Chelikani P, Fita I, and Loewen P 2004. Diversity of structures and properties among catalases. *Cell Mol. Life Sci*. 61(2): 192–208.

Christen Y, 2000. Oxidative stress and Alzheimer disease. *Am. J. Clin. Nutr.* 71(2): 621S–629S.

Cook NR, Albert CM, and Gaziano JM 2007. A randomized factorial trial of vitamins C and E and beta carotene in the secondary prevention of cardiovascular events in women: results from the women's antioxidant cardiovascular study. *Arch. Intern. Med*. 167(15): 1610–8.

Cookson M, and Shaw P 1999. Oxidative stress and motor neurone disease. *Brain Pathol* 9(1): 165–86.

Davì G, Falco A, and Patrono C 2005. Lipid peroxidation in diabetes mellitus. *Antioxid Redox Signal* 7(1–2): 256–68.

Davies K, 1995. "Oxidative stress: the paradox of aerobic life". *Biochem. Soc. Symp.* 61: 1–31.

Ercal I, Sayed H, *et al*. 2001. Prominent free radical scavenging activity of tannic acid in lead induced oxidative stress in experimental mice. *Toxicol. Ind. Health* 22: 157–163.

Evans M and Co. 1998. Risk factors for excess phytates in diet: An overview. www.diagnosme.com/cond/c21360.html.

Fajardo-Lirai, Henning SM, Lee HW, Go VLW, and Heber D 2002. Department Family Environmental Sciences/Nutrition, Dietetics & Food Science, California State University, Northridge and UCLA Center for Human Nutrition, Session 46C, Annual meeting of Food Expo, Anaheim.

Frei B, 2009. "Controversy: What are the true biological functions of superfruit antioxidants? ".http://www.npicenter.com/anm/templates/newsATemp.aspx?articleid=23667&zoneid=273.

Giugliano D, Ceriello A, and Paolisso G 1996. Oxidative stress and diabetic vascular complications. *Diabetes Care* 19(3): 257–67.

Graf E, Empson KL, and Eaton JW 1987. Phytic acid. A natural antioxidant. *The Journal of Biological Chemistry*, 262: 11647–11650.

Hitchon C, and El-Gabalawy H 2004. Oxidation in rheumatoid arthritis. *Arthritis Res. Ther.* 6(6): 65–78.

Imlay J, 2003. Pathways of oxidative damage. *Annu. Rev Microbiol.* 57: 395–418.

Jang M, Cai L, Udeani GO, *et al.* 1997. Cancer chemo preventive activity of resveratrol, a natural product derived from grapes". *Science* 275(5297): 218–20.

Jiménez-Monreal AM, García-Diz L, Martínez-Tomé M, Mariscal M, and Murcia MA 2009. Influence of cooking methods on antioxidant activity of vegetables. *Journal of Food Science* 74(3): H97–H103.

Johnson F, and Giulivi C 2005. Superoxide dismutases and their impact upon human health. *Mol. Aspects Med.* 26(4–5): 340–52.

Kopke RD, Jackson RL, Coleman JK, Liu J, Bielefeld EC, and Balough BJ 2007. NAC for noise: from the bench top to the clinic. *Hear. Res.* 226(1–2): 114–25.

Lirai S, Henning H, Lee V, *et al.* 2002. Beneficial health effects of polyphenol antioxidants in green tea blends. Proc Ann meeting of Food Expo, Anaheim, Ca, Dept. of Diatetics and Food Sc, California state Univ.

Lotito SB, and Frei B 2006. Consumption of flavonoid-rich foods and increased plasma antioxidant capacity in humans: cause, consequence, or epiphenomenon? *Free Radic. Biol. Med.* 41(12): 1727–46.

Mcbrien D, and Slater T 1992. Antitumor and antioxidant activity of naturally occurring isothiocyanates. Academic press, London, pp. 173–195.

Mei Y, Wei D, and Liu J 2005. Reversal of multidrug resistance in KB cells with tea polyphenol antioxidant capacity. *Cancer Biol. Ther.* 4(4): 468–73.

Minihane A, and Gerald R 2002. Iron absorption and the iron binding and antioxidant properties of phytic acid. *International Journal of Food Science and Technology* 37: 741–748.

Muldoon MF, and Kritchevsky SB 1996. Flavonoids and heart disease. *BMJ* 312(7029): 458–9.

Nozik-Grayck E, Suliman H, and Piantadosi C 2005. Extracellular superoxide dismutase. *Int. J. Biochem. Cell Biol.* 37(12): 2466–71.

Nunomura A, Castellani R, Zhu X, Moreira P, Perry G, and Smith M 2006. "Involvement of oxidative stress in Alzheimer disease". *J. Neuropathol. Exp. Neurol.* 65(7): 631–41.

Rhee SG 2006. "Cell signaling. H_2O_2, a necessary evil for cell signaling". *Science* 312(5782): 1882–3.

RRI (Report of the Rowett Research Institute) 1995. Free radicals, antioxidants and disease.

Serafini M, Laranjinha JA, Almeida LM, and Maiani G 2000. Inhibition of human LDL lipid peroxidation by phenol-rich beverages and their impact on plasma total antioxidant capacity in humans. *J. Nutr. Biochem.* (11–12): 585–590.

Sies H, 1997. Oxidative stress: oxidants and antioxidants. *Exp Physiol.* 82(2): 291–5.

Slater V, and Tolonen M 1990. Free radicals and antioxidant micronutrients. *Proc. Soc. Exp. Biol. Med.* 193: 16–22.

Stanner SA, Hughes J, Kelly CN, and Buttriss J 2004. A review of the epidemiological evidence for the 'antioxidant hypothesis. *Public Health Nutr.* 7(3): 407–22.

Van Gaal L, Mertens I, and De Block C 2006. Mechanisms linking obesity with cardiovascular disease. *Nature* 444(7121): 875–80.

Vertuani S, Angusti A, and Manfredini S 2004. The antioxidants and pro-antioxidants network: an overview. *Curr. Pharm. Des* 10(14): 1677–94.

Virgili F, and Marino M 2008. Regulation of cellular signals from nutritional molecules: a specific role for phytochemicals, beyond antioxidant activity. *Free Radical Biology & Medicine* 45(9): 1205–16.

Williams RJ, Spencer JP, and Rice-Evans C 2004. Flavonoids: antioxidants or signalling molecules?. *Free Radical Biology & Medicine* 36(7): 838–49.

Wood-Kaczmar A, Gandhi S, and Wood N 2006. Understanding the molecular causes of Parkinson's disease. *Trends Mol. Med.* 12(11): 521–8.

5

Factors Influencing Antioxidant Activity of Fruits and Vegetables

"Now we are entering an era whereby the quality of food must be raised by maintaining or improving not only typical attributes for food, such as microbiological or toxicological safety, nutritional value, sensory properties (such as taste, flavor, texture, appearance and color), but also its health promoting property *viz*. Antioxidant capacity" (Lerici, 1998).

In order to evaluate the healthiness of raw food and to optimize processing conditions, the health promoting capacity and changes in it during storage and/or processing are essential to be measured.

Recent studies emphasize the usage of fruits and vegetables as rich sources of antioxidant micronutrients. Due to the seasonal nature, for many of the fruits, certain processing techniques such as drying,

Reported studies on antioxidant activities of fruits and vegetables

- High ORAC in dark green cruciferous vegetables and citrus fruits (Fergusson *et al*, 1999, Vinson *et al*, 1999)
- High ORAC in brussels sprouts, spinach, kale and dark grapes (Arts *et al*, 2000, Szeto *et al*, 2002)
- High SOSA, FICA and polyphenol content in *Garcinia indica* (Yamaguchi *et al*, 2000)
- High ITBARS in 11 fruits, 3 GLVs and 3 cereals (NIN Annual report 1997-98)
- High ITBARS and polyphenols in gooseberry, black carrots, kachnar and ginger (Kaur *et al*, 2002)

Plate 28

canning, marmalade and jam preparations have been developed to facilitate the consumption of the same round the year, even in the absence of season of that particular food commodity. Although extensive usages of the same are prevalent, the losses in the antioxidant and micronutrient quality due to processing of the foods are less taken into account.

Phytochemicals are a heterogeneous group of molecules with protective function on human health, when their dietary intake is significant. The functional properties are antioxidant activity, modulation of detoxification enzymes, stimulation of the immune system, decrease of platelet aggregation and modulation of hormone metabolism. Glucosinolates and group of polyphenols, including the main category of flavonoids, have been reported widely. Due to their weak estrogenic activity, isoflavones are also included. Numerous factors can affect the antioxidant and micronutrient content and their bioavailability in foods. These factors include environmental conditions and industrial or domestic processing. The bioavailability of antioxidants and micronutrients can be further be influenced by intrinsic factors in food and/or in human body. In general the phytochemicals are little absorbed, largely metabolized and rapidly eliminated. For this reason

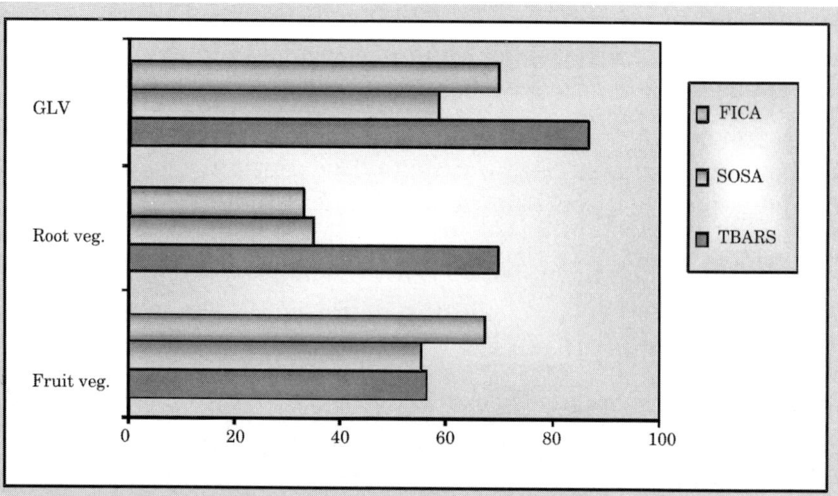

Paired *t* values for antioxidant indices of the differences between uncooked and cooked fruit-root vegetables and GLV were highly significant.

Cooking losses for the antioxidant indices in vegetables

Plate 29

it is advisable that their consumption is constant in the time to maintain high concentrations of metabolites in the blood (Carratù and Sanzini, 2005). Plates 28-38 depict the results of authors experiments.

Multiple regression equations for antioxidant indices (Tarwadi and Agte, 2007)

Antioxidant capacity	*Cooked GLV (n = 30)*	*Adjusted R^2*	*Significance*
ITBARS	0.621–1.219* Zn ± 2.85* Cu–0.00127* ß-Carotene	0.35	F = 4.2, p = 0.023
SOSA	–5.477 ± 350.306* Se ± 0.22* vit C	0.487	F = 9.55, p = 0.002
FICA	37.187–143.698* Zn–385.84* Se ± 852* thiamine	0.32	
Other cooked vegetables (n = 27)			
ITBARS	–0.134 ± 0.76* Cu ± 0.0013* polyphenols ± 0.03* vit C	0.51	F = 10.0, p = 0.0001
SOSA	16.183 ± 33.288* Cu	0.10	F = 3.57, p = 0.07
FICA	10.939 ± 3.019* Mn	0.21	F = 8.1, p = 0.009

Values of nutrients expressed per 100 g fresh weight were used for analysis

Plate 30

AGRONOMIC PRACTICES

The survey of existing literature comparing nutrient content of organic and conventional crops using statistical methods has been done to identify significant differences and trends in the data (Worthington, 2001). Organic crops contained significantly more vitamin C, iron, magnesium, and phosphorus and significantly less nitrates than conventional crops. There were non-significant trends showing less protein but of a better quality and a higher content of nutritionally significant minerals with lower amounts of some heavy metals in organic crops compared to conventional ones. Regular consumption of tomatoes has been associated with decreased risk of chronic degenerative diseases. Epidemiological findings confirm the observed health effects are due to the presence of different antioxidant molecules such as carotenoids, particularly lycopene, ascorbic acid, vitamin E and phenol compounds, particularly flavonoids (Frusciante *et al.*, 2007). Replicated field trials at three matched farm pairs in southern and central Taiwan were established in October 2004 and 2005 to compare fruit quality and nutritional parameters of tomatoes grown on-farm under organic versus conventional management systems in tropical and subtropical environments. Farm management skills combined with site-specific effects contributed to high lycopene levels, and the choice of variety significantly influenced the content of bioactive compounds, particularly ascorbic acid and total phenolics (Juroszek *et al.*, 2009).

Leafy vegetables are highly perishable and their shelf life depends on duration and conditions of storage. A low cost storage structure was used to extend the shelf life of amaranth and fenugreek and their quality was evaluated on the basis of retention of beta-carotene, ascorbic acid and chlorophyll during storage (Negi and Roy, 2003). Losses of beta-carotene were reported from 46.5 to 85.0% for amaranth and 24.0 to 73.0% for fenugreek depending on duration and conditions of storage. Similarly ascorbic acid retention varied from 9–32% for amaranth and 23–80% for fenugreek. Results showed that the degradation of quality parameters was faster at ambient conditions and packaging of leaves in low density polyethylene bags was beneficial in improving shelf life and nutritive value. Low cost storage structure was similar to low temperature storage for retention of beta-carotene, ascorbic acid, chlorophyll content and enhancement of shelf life.

COOKING METHODS

The influence of home cooking methods (boiling, microwaving, pressure-cooking, griddling, frying, and baking) on the antioxidant activity of vegetables was evaluated by Jiménez-Monreal *et al.* (2009) for 20 locally available vegetables, using different antioxidant activity assays (lipoperoxyl and hydroxyl radicals scavenging and TEAC). Artichoke was the only vegetable showing very high scavenging-lipoperoxyl radical capacity in all the cooking methods. Beetroot and green bean retained their antioxidant activity after most cooking treatments. In fact, celery increased its antioxidant capacity in all the cooking methods, except boiling when it lost 14%. On the other hand, highest losses of lipoperoxyl scavenging capacity were observed in cauliflower after boiling and microwaving, pea after boiling, and zucchini after boiling and frying. Swiss chard and pepper lost hydroxyl scavenging capacity in all the processes. Analysis of the ABTS radical scavenging capacity of the different vegetables showed that the highest losses occurred in garlic with all the methods, except microwaving. Among the vegetables that increased their TEAC values were green bean, celery, and carrot after all cooking methods (except green bean after boiling). These vegetables showed a low ABTS radical scavenging capacity. According to the method of analysis chosen, griddling, microwave cooking, and baking alternately had lowest losses, while pressure-cooking and boiling lead to the greatest losses; frying occupies an intermediate position.

Carotenoids contribute to the beneficial effects of fruits and vegetables consumption; however, the bioavailability of these compounds from fresh or processed foods is not well established. Carotenoid mass-balance calculations using ileostomy subjects indicated that 65.1 +/- 7.4% of the beta-carotene was absorbed from cooked pureed carrot meals, *vs*. 41.4 +/-7.4% from raw, chopped carrot meals (Linvy, 2003).

The Maillard reaction occurs widely in food and biological systems. A review for the relation between the Maillard reaction and food processing, particularly its contribution to flavor formation, antioxidative effects, desmutagenic activity and the improvement of protein functional properties has been reported. Proteins modified by glucose, and melanoidins are important components of foodstuffs while the reactions of amino acids or peptides with glucose or dicarbonyl compounds produce various kinds of flavor components. Melanoidins and Amadori rearrangement products play an important part in providing antioxidative effects, both *in vitro* and *in vivo*. Melanoidins also exhibit desmutagenic activity against carcinogenic compounds. Protein-polysaccharide conjugates, prepared by Maillard reaction at mild conditions, increase the emulsifying activity, as well as antioxidative and antimicrobial effects of the original proteins (Chuyen, 1998).

INDUSTRIAL PROCESSING

Citrus fruits and juices are rich in a number of bioactive compounds. Their antioxidant activity and related benefits derive not only from vitamin C but also from flavonoids. During juice processing, temperature and oxygen are the main factors responsible for vitamin C losses. Processed juices without heat treatment retain higher levels of vitamin C, but economic factors apparently delay the use of such methods in the citrus industry. Regarding packing material, vitamin C in fruit juice is quite stable when stored in metal or glass containers, whereas juice stored in plastic bottles has a much shorter shelf-life (Marti *et al.*, 2009).

Epidemiological studies suggest the consumption of a flavonoids rich diet such as onion, the richest and most common source, of quercetin might decrease the risk of degenerative changes and certain diseases. Quercetin is present in onion mainly as glycosides, of which the distribution within the onion bulb changes in onion processing. After ingestion, quercetin is reported to undergo extensive metabolism and microbial action resulting in its altered or degraded structure; therefore, most of the effects shown in *in vitro* experiments with the pure compound cannot be directly extrapolated to *in vivo* systems (Nemeth and Piskula, 2007).

Berries and nuts, are rich sources of ellagitannins and ellagic acid, a hydrolytic product of ellagitannins (ETs). These secondary metabolites give the characteristic taste, and play an important role in food processing. Pomegranates, and walnuts are also important sources of ETs. ET concentrations of some products (pomegranate, muscadine grape and berries juices, and wines) increase after processing (Bakkalbasi *et al.*, 2009).

Fats impart taste and texture to the product, however, it is susceptible to oxidation resulting in the development of rancidity and off-flavor. Discovery of synthetic antioxidants has revolutionized the use of antioxidants in food. The effect of these antioxidants in bakery products were reviewed and found to be effective in enhancing the shelf life. Further, animal experimental studies have shown that some of the synthetic antioxidants had toxigenic, mutagenic, and carcinogenic effects. Hence there is an increasing demand for the use of natural antioxidants in foods, especially in bakery products. Some of the natural antioxidants like alpha-tocopherol, beta-carotene, and ascorbic acid are already used in bakery products. These natural antioxidants are effective in enhancing the shelf life of bakery products but not to the extent of synthetic antioxidants. Baking processing steps may lower the antioxidative activity but techniques such as encapsulation of antioxidants can retain their activity. Antioxidative activity of garcinia, curcumin, vanillins, and mint were reviewed but studies on their role in bakery products were limited or very few. A wide scope for study under this direction in depth, is indicated. (Nandita and Prabhasankar, 2009).

Natural lipids are principally esters of long chain fatty acids, phospholipids and sterols, consumed as food and added as functional ingredients in many processed foods. However, they are also the most chemically unstable food components. Lipids readily undergo free-radical chain reactions that not only deteriorate the lipids but also produce oxidative fragments, some of which are volatile and are perceived as the off-flavors of rancidity, degrade proteins, vitamins and pigments and cross-link lipids and other macromolecules into non-nutritive

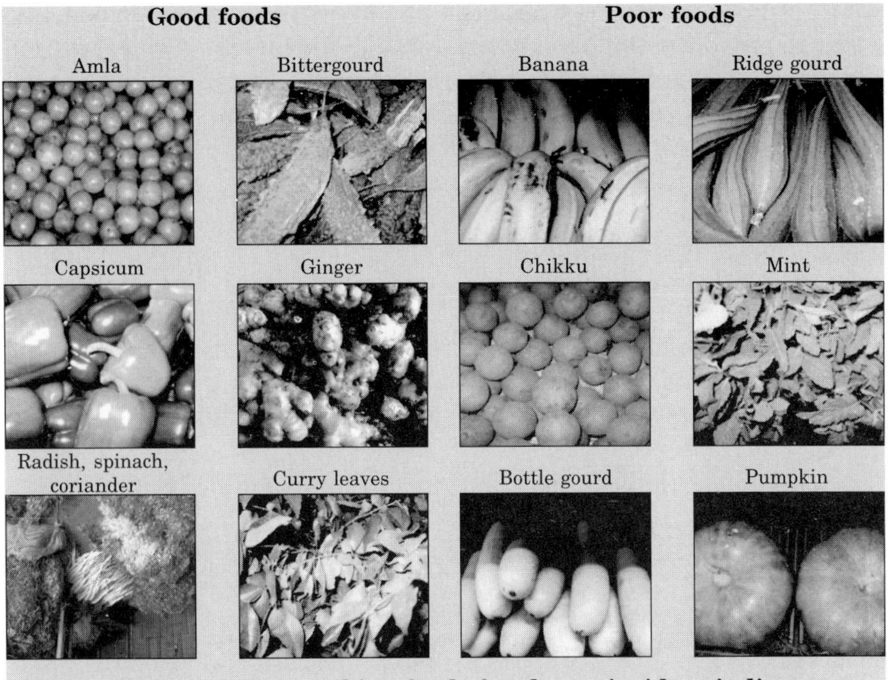

Good and poor ranking foods for the antioxidant indices

Plate 31

polymers. The effects of raw product selection, harvesting, storage, refining, manufacturing and distribution, on the quality of lipids in the final commodity are significant. Certain key variables now known to influence oxidative processes can be targeted to increase food lipid stability during and after processing. Retention of or addition of exogenous antioxidants is a well-known consideration, but the presence and activity of catalysts, the integrity of tissues and cells, the quantity of polyunsaturated lipids and the structural properties of the final food product, including total surface area of lipids, and the nature of surfactant materials all play important roles in final product stability (German, 1999).

The intake of flavonoids on quality and quantity depends on dietary habits and a widespread presence of quercetin in the diet makes this compound one of the key factors. Even after being metabolized it may still affect the redox balance by inducing antioxidative and detoxifying enzymes or compounds which may be involved in sustaining homeostasis (Nemeth and Piskula, 2007).

Consumption of berries has been linked with diverse health benefits, such as prevention of stroke, age-related degenerative diseases and cancer. Some berry constituents have cancer preventive actions on chemically induced tumors *in vivo* and cancer suppressive effects in *in vitro* studies. Many of these effects were due to specific berry phytochemicals with high antioxidative potential that could contribute to, or enhance by induction, the endogenous antioxidant properties of living cells or organisms. Manufacturers and the consumers of berry products need more comprehensive and accurate information on the type and level of health benefits expected from different products. The choice of the chemical or biological test that best predicts specific health benefits of berries is crucial to provide targets for berry breeding programmes or to improve processing methods (Juraniae and Zizak, 2005).

Antioxidant capacity and polyphenols in fresh fruits as well as uncooked and cooked vegetables

Food class	*ITBARS mM vitamin E eq./100g*	*SOSA mM Tannic acid eq./100g*	*FICA mM EDTA eq./100g*	*Polyphenols mg /100g*
Fruit veg. cooked	0.19 ± 0.25	19.83 ± 10.4	14.39 ± 3.8	134.6 ± 48.21
Root veg. cooked	0.44 ± 0.20	21.2 ± 12.4	17.23 ± 9.64	232.1 ± 44.03
GLV cooked	0.40 ± 0.10	18.3 ± 10.16	23.5 ± 14.3	94.5 ± 30.1
Fruits (fresh)	0.44 ± 0.23	33.3 ± 15.8	35.07 ± 15.2	179.7 ± 311.4
Fruit veg. uncooked	0.49 ± 0.21	40.7 ± 15.6	41.6 ± 14.9	143.6 ± 60
Root veg. uncooked	0.69 ± 0.21	36.2 ± 18.7	35.51 ± 14.75	251.4 ± 107.3
GLV uncooked	0.73 ± 0.23	31.7 ± 16.8	34.2 ± 17.3	111 ± 45.8

Plate 32

The carotenoid compositions of foods vary both qualitatively and quantitatively. For a given food, compositional variability occurs due to stage of maturity, variety or cultivar, climate or season, part of the plant consumed, production practices, post-harvest handling, processing and storage of food. During processing, isomerization of trans-forms (the usual configuration in nature) to the cis-forms occurs, with consequent alteration of their' bioavailability and biological activity. Isomerization is promoted by light, heat and acids. The major cause of carotenoid loss during processing and storage of food is enzymatic or non-enzymatic oxidation of the highly unsaturated carotenoid molecules. The extent of damage depends on the presence of oxygen, metals, enzymes, unsaturated lipids, prooxidants, antioxidants; exposure to light; type and physical state of the carotenoids present; severity and duration of processing; packaging material; storage conditions. Therefore, retention of carotenoids has been the major concern in the preparation, processing and storage of foods. Further, in recent years the effect of processing on bioavailability has been in focus. More than a century after their discovery, carotenoids continue to be intensely investigated in various areas. An overview of current knowledge in Food Science and Technology, with bearing on the role of carotenoids in human health has been given by Rodriguez-Amaya (2003).

Inhibition of lipid peroxidation as mM vitamin E equivalents/100g in various fruits	
0.1–0.2	Big banana, Chikku, Lemon, Musk melon, Water melon
0.2–0.3	Ziziphus, Pineapple, Carissa, Plum, Strawberry, Custard apple, Green tamarind
0.3–0.4	Pomegranate, Ramphal (bullock's heart), Ripe mango, Wood apple, Yellow raisins
0.4–0.5	Raisins black, Cashew fruit
0.5–0.6	Red tamarind, Yellow zizyphus, Sweet lime, Small Banana
0.6–0.7	Big amla, Zizhphus small, Orange, Rose apple, Dry and Fresh dates, apple, Water chestnut
0.7–0.8	Bel fruit, Dry figs, Kokum

Plate 33

Tocopherols are a class of phenolic antioxidants which can inhibit lipid autoxidation by scavenging free radicals and by reacting with singlet oxygen. In vegetable oils alpha-tocopherol prevents the effects of singlet oxygen during sensitized photoxidation. After processing of

Super oxide scavenging activity as nM of EDTA equivalents/100g in various fruits	
0–10	Small banana
10–20	Chikku, Water melon, Pomegranate, Big banana, Musk melon, Yellow raisins, Small zizyphus, Orange, Big amla, Carissa
20–30	Strawberry, Apple, Ramphal, Plums, Wood apple, Pineapple
30–40	Papaya, Custard apple, Guava tamarind, Big zizyphus, Yellow zizyphus, Black raisins
40–50	Ripe mango, Kokum, Lemon, Rose apple, Sweet lime, Small amla
50–60	Cashew fruit, Red tamarind, Fresh dates
60–70	Dry figs, Water chestnut, Dry dates
70–80	Bel fruit

Plate 34

Fe^{+2} chelation activity as mM EDTA equivalents/100g in various fruits (Tarwadi and Agte, 2007)

0–10	Big and small banana
10–20	Ripe mango, Chikku, Water melon, Strawberry, Carissa
20–30	Musk melon, Wood apple, Plum, Sweet lime, Pomegranate
30–40	Orange, Ramphal, Small/big/yellow zizyphus, Tamarind, Kokum fruit
40–50	Papaya, Dry dates, Lemon, Raisins black, Custard apple, Pineapple, Fresh dates, Guava, Rose apple, Dry figs. Cashew fruit
50–60	Dry figs, Water chestnut, Dry dates
60–70	Big amla, Bel fruit

Plate 35

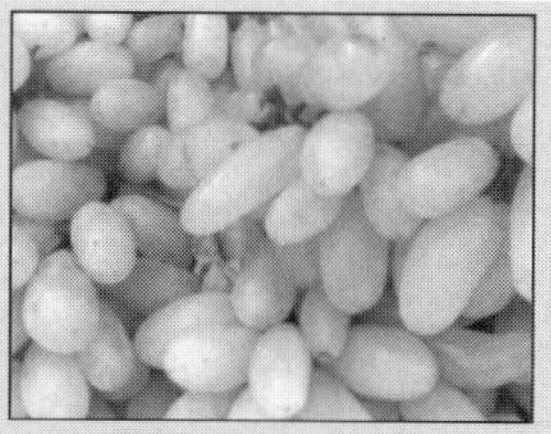

Green grapes

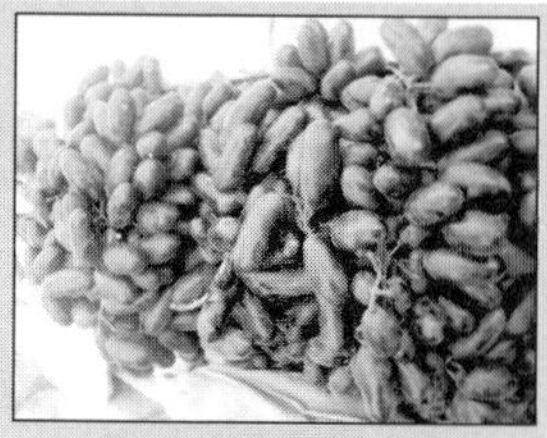

Purple grapes

- Contain flavonoids like Catechin and Resveratrol
- Anthocyanins from grape rinds exhibit anti-tumor effect
- Anti-inflammatory and anti-cancer activity
- Free radical scavenging activity

Antioxidant and micronutrient potential of grapes

Plate 36

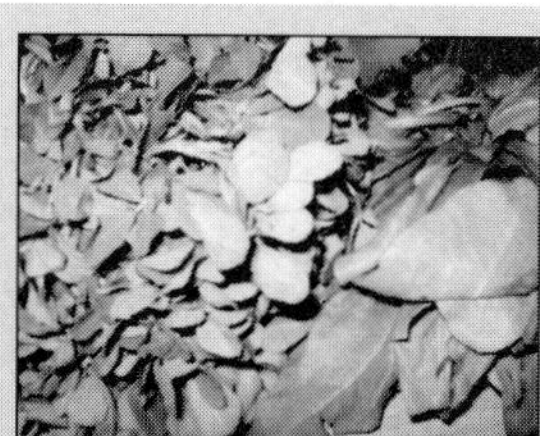

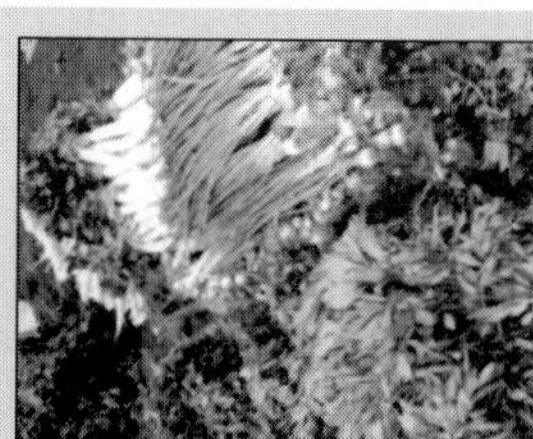

Antioxidants	*GLV*	*Other Veg.*	*Fruits*	*Cereals*	*Legumes*
Vitamin C (mg %)	5 – 281	0 – 137	0 – 212	0	0 – 3
α carotene (μg %)	250 – 14190	0 – 1890	0 – 2743	0 – 132	0 – 469
Zinc (mg %)	0.08 – 3.44	0.11 – 2.29	0.03 – 0.82	1.3 – 3.1	0.9 – 6.1
Copper (mg %)	0.04 – 2.32	0.02 – 0.29	0.03 – 0.6	0.07 – 1.4	0.39 – 1.87
Iron (mg %)	0.8 – 38.5	0.5 – 7.4	2.7 – 10.4	0.7 – 8.0	2.7 – 10.4

Why Green Leafy Vegetables? (Agte *et al.*, 2000)

Plate 37

Potential of commonly consumed green leafy vegetables for their antioxidant capacity and their linkage with micronutrient profile (Tarwadi and Agte, 2003)
• There is a large variability in different GLVs for their antioxidant capacities. • Cooking losses in GLV for three indices are high (26%–41%) and significant ($p < 0.001$). • Top ranking GLVs for the antioxidant indices in both cooked and cooked states are: Tamarind, Fenugreek, Cauliflower, Coriander, Radish, Spinach, Drumstick, Green amaranthus gogu, Curry leaves.

Plate 38

vegetable oils, about 60–70% of the tocopherols are retained in the oil. Tocopherol levels in processed vegetable oils, is generally above the optimum range for antioxidant activity. On the other hand, beta-carotene is almost completely removed during processing of vegetable oils. For antioxidant purposes, both beta-carotene and ascorbic acid must be added to vegetable oils after deodorization (Frankel, 1989).

Nutraceuticals have potent biological actions. Their use is increasing drastically, and there is growing evidence of clinical benefits. No medicinal products are completely safe and their risks have to be characterized and controlled. Imposing pharmaceutical levels of control and regulation would increase costs and reduce patient access to new products, but the evidence is compelling that closer monitoring of raw materials, processing and formulation will be required to maximize the benefits and minimize the risks (Hardy *et al.*, 2003).

Effect of processing on antioxidant capacity in selected fruits (authors experiments)

It is well known that the micronutrient contents, mainly vitamins like vitamin C, beta-carotene, riboflavin and thiamine being heat-labile, gets destroyed if any methods involving use of heat or exposure to oxygen are adapted for processing. It is also generally recognized, but poorly investigated, that storage as well as processing can negatively affect the original antioxidant properties of foods (Korver, 1997). The antioxidant potential in any food/food product is mainly conferred by the presence of the antioxidant vitamins or polyphenols that may be lost upon processing. In fact, food processing, especially if heat treatment based, can result in undesired reactions, mostly of a chemical nature. For instance, oxidation can occur as the consequence of antioxidants and vitamins depletion. On the other hand, heating can also induce the formation of compounds with new antioxidant properties, as occurs during the development of the Maillard reaction in which a reducing sugar reacts with amino groups. Properties of Maillard reaction products (MRPs) in food processing and preservation can positively or negatively affect nutritional and sensorial properties, and shelf life of the products (Elizalde *et al.*, 1991; Lerici *et al.*, 1994).

There is little data available about changes in the antioxidant loss due to processing and/or storage on the simultaneous formation of MRPs with antioxidant properties following heat treatment (Nicoli *et al.*, 1997). Although natural antioxidants can be lost during heating, the overall antioxidant properties of food can be maintained or enhanced by the formation of new antioxidants (Nicoli *et al.*, 1997). In tomato juice, the heating caused an increase in its antioxidant potential, even if short heat treatment caused an initial reduction in the original antioxidant property, probably due to formation in the early stages of the Maillard Reaction of intermediate compounds with pro-oxidant activity (Lerici *et al.*, 1996). Analysis of coffee beverages confirmed that total antioxidant properties were greatly increased with degree of roasting (Nicoli *et al.*, 1997).

It remains to be seen if the denaturation of fruits leads to changes in the antioxidant potential. The necessary measuring systems are the lipid oxidation tests for measurement of overall antioxidant activity and radical scavenging capacity. In the light of this background, an exercise was undertaken with an aim to assess the antioxidant capacities as ITBARS and FICA, as well as contents of micronutrients mainly vitamin C and beta-carotene in bael fruit, guava and Indian gooseberry (amla), that elicited promising antioxidant potential among the screened fruits. The fruits selected were guava, bael fruit and gooseberry that manifested topmost antioxidant potential among the fruits previously screened by us. The fruits were subjected to various methods of drying.

METHODS

The dehydration methods selected were oven drying, sun drying, air-drying and freeze-drying. The dehydrated samples were analysed for ITBARS, FICA, contents of ascorbic acid and beta-carotene using previously described assays.

- *Sun-drying technique*: The fruits were cut into pieces (2 mm × 2 mm × 2 mm each) and allowed to dry under direct sunlight till complete dryness was achieved.

- *Oven-drying technique*: The samples were kept in oven at 45°C till all the moisture was removed. The temperature was purposely kept lower to avoid charring of fruits.
- *Air-drying technique*: The fruits were allowed to get dehydrated at room temperature by leaving in open air till complete dryness.
- *Freeze-drying technique*: The samples were lyophilized at –70°C for 30 min, till all the moisture was removed.

Losses in the antioxidant activities and micronutrients upon dehydration

The antioxidant micronutrient potential of fruits prior to drying can be seen from Table 5.1.

Table 5.1: Antioxidant micronutrient potential of fruits prior to drying

Fruit	*ITBARS mM vit E/100 g*	*FICA mM EDTA/100 g*	*Ascorbic acid mg/100 g*	*β-carotene μg/100 g*
Guava	0.92	47.8	148.0	98.0
Bael-fruit	0.74	62.0	12.0	28.0
Gooseberry	0.63	61.6	445.0	16.0

The % loss in the ITBARS activity, FICA, ascorbic acid and beta-carotene for guava, bael-fruit and gooseberry observed for the different methods of drying can be visualized from Tables 5.2–5.5.

Sun drying of fruits resulted in maximum loss for all the measured indices (Table 2). For guava, retention of ITBARS and ascorbic acid was negligible; FICA and ascorbic acid was only 10%. Bael fruit lost nearly all the ITBARS activity and could hardly retain 10% of FICA, ascorbic acid and beta-carotene. Gooseberry (amla) could perform relatively better by being able to retain 27.2% of ITBARS and 25% ascorbic acid, 50% of FICA and 31.3% beta-carotene.

Table 5.2: Loss (%) observed for sun-drying method

Fruit	*ITBARS mM vit E/100 g*	*FICA mM EDTA/100 g*	*Ascorbic acid mg/100 g*	*β-carotene μg/100 g*
Guava	96.0	86.5	98.0	86.5
Bael-fruit	97.0	90.3	90.0	92.8
Gooseberry	72.8	50.0	75.0	68.7

The observations for oven-drying and air-drying methods were somewhat analogous (Tables 5.3 and 5.4). The differences of the values between the two drying methods were non significant ($p>0.05$). Guava could retain about 27.2 and 28.7% ITBARS activity, 43.5 and 48% FICA. The loss in ascorbic acid was quite high with only 12% being retained after oven-drying and 22% after air-drying. Losses for beta-carotene were also high with only 36% and 29% retention following oven and air-drying respectively. The retention in bael fruit were also low *viz.* 55.4% after oven drying and 63.5% after air-drying of the initial ITBARS. For FICA, 31.5% and 43% oven and air-drying respectively. Similarly for ascorbic acid values of retention were 32% and 43% and for beta-carotene 54% and 71.4%. Gooseberry could retain 57% ITBARS and 48% FICA with both drying methods. Ascorbic acid retentions were drastically low *i.e.* 18% and 11%. Further, only 25% and 34.7% of beta-carotene remained in gooseberry after oven drying and air-drying.

Table 5.3: Loss (%) observed for oven-drying method

Fruit	*ITBARS mM vit E/100 g*	*FICA mM EDTA/100 g*	*Ascorbic acid mg/100 g*	*β-carotene µg/100 g*
Guava	72.8	56.5	88.0	64.0
Bael-fruit	44.6	68.5	68.0	46.0
Gooseberry	43.0	52.0	82.0	75.0

Table 5.4: Loss (%) observed for air-drying method

Fruit	*ITBARS mM vit E/100 g*	*FICA mM EDTA/100 g*	*Ascorbic acid mg/100 g*	*β-carotene µg/100 g*
Guava	71.3	52.0	78.0	71.0
Bael-fruit	36.5	57.0	57.0	28.6
Gooseberry	36.0	47.0	89.0	64.3

Freeze drying method showed maximum retention for all the parameters as expected (Table 5.5). Bael fruit and gooseberry showed higher retention than guava by all the methods for all the parameters. Among all the 4 indices, losses of ascorbic acid were highest for the 3 fruits, though lowest loss was seen for the freeze-drying technique. Losses for beta-carotene were found to be least by air-drying method.

Table 5.5: Loss (%) observed for freeze-drying method

Fruit	*ITBARS mM vit E/100 g*	*FICA mM EDTA/100 g*	*Ascorbic acid mg/100 g*	*β-carotene μg/100 g*
Guava	56.5	46.4	59.0	65.0
Bael-fruit	37.8	38.0	40.0	45.7
Gooseberry	50.0	46.2	58.5	75.0

Antioxidant micronutrient potential of some processed products

The processed marketed products of gooseberry are quite popular in India and are habitually consumed. Since gooseberry was a merit fruit for the antioxidant potential, ascorbic acid and polyphenols, it was of interest to look into the same parameters among the processed marketed products of gooseberry as well. The antioxidant micronutrient potential and contents of polyphenols in some popular products of gooseberry have been stated in Table 5.6.

Table 5.6: Antioxidant and micronutrient contents of gooseberry products

Product	*ITBARS mM vit E/ 100 g*	*FICA mM EDTA/ 100 g*	*Ascorbic acid mg/ 100 g*	*β-carotene μg/ 100 g*	*Polyphenols mg/ 100 g*
Muravla	0.33	10.21	58.32	4	1123
Amla candy	0.41	8.33	21.23	4	988
Amla meva	0.48	21.64	64.49	2	1011
Pachak amla	0.31	15.85	30.36	5	848
Sharbat	0.44	20.21	28.86	7	599
Jam	0.31	11.15	27.88	1	747
Amla supari	0.19	12.33	27.48	0	1318
Amla pickle	0.45	17.85	63.71	5	879
Chyawanprash	0.20	20.26	12.12	2	1029

Muravla (gooseberry in sugar syrup) is a concoction of grated amla with sugar having a longer lasting shelf life. Candy (dried sweetened amla), pachak amla (grated salted amla), supari (dried salted amla), meva (grated dried sweetened amla), sharbat (amla juice concentrate), jam, regular amla pickle and chyawanprash (an Ayurvedic tonic) are very popular and do not need much prologue. As compared to fresh gooseberry (Table 5.1), ITBARS were highest in meva followed by amla pickle and lowest in supari and chyawanprash. FICA was found to be similar and less than one-third of the fresh gooseberry values in meva, sharbat and chyanprash and lowest in candy indicating significant processing losses ($p<0.001$).

Although gooseberry has highest ascorbic acid content, the losses in the content of ascorbic acid were 86% to 97% and were significantly high for all the processed products ($p<0.001$). Even then, among the products, meva could retain highest ascorbic acid (64.5 mg %) followed by pickle (63.7%). Surprisingly, chyawanprash, which is widely propagated for high contents of ascorbic acid, was found to be containing least amounts of ascorbic acid.

The loss in the beta-carotene contents was not significant ($p>0.05$), because gooseberry is not a promising source of beta-carotene. Among the processed products, sharbat retained 7 µg% beta-carotene, probably because of no heat treatment being involved in the processing. The polyphenols in fresh amla was found to be highest among all the fruits (1324 mg %), however, among the products, polyphenols were found to be retained maximum in supari, followed by muravla; the loss being marginally significant ($p<0.05$).

In conclusion, the methods adopted for the dehydration of fruits were chosen based on routine household methods practiced and confirmed significant losses in the antioxidant activities; nevertheless yet other more suitable methods for better retention of antioxidant potential in the processed products are required to be explored in order to further combine quality with health benefits. Further improvement in the stages concerned with the processes involved in the food sequence such as production, storage, packaging, etc. might prove to be further useful in order to trail total quality of foods.

REFERENCES

Bakkalbasi E, Mentes O, and Artik N 2009. Food ellagitannins-occurrence, effects of processing and storage. *Crit. Rev. Food Sci. Nutr.* 49(3): 283–98.

Carratù B, and Sanzini E 2005. Biologically-active phytochemicals in vegetable food *Ann. Ist Super Sanita*. 41(1): 7–16.

Chuyen NV, 1998. Maillard reaction and food processing. Application aspects. *Adv. Exp. Med. Biol.* 434: 213–35.

Elizalde B, Dalla M, and Lerici C 1991. Effect of maillard reaction volatile products on lipid oxidation. *J. Am. Oil. Chem. Soc.* 68: 758–762.

Frankel EN, 1989. The antioxidant and nutritional effects of tocopherols, ascorbic acid and beta-carotene in relation to processing of edible oils. *Bibl. Nutr. Dieta.* 43: 297–312.

Frusciante L, Carli P, Ercolano R, Pernice R, Di Matteo A, Fogliano V, and Pellegrini N, 2007. Antioxidant nutritional quality of tomato. *Mol. Nutr. Food Res.* 5(15): 609–17.

German JB, 1999. Food processing and lipid oxidation. *Adv. Exp. Med. Biol.* 459: 23–50.

Hardy G, Hardy I, and Ball PA 2003. Nutraceuticals—a pharmaceutical viewpoint: part II. *Curr. Opin. Clin. Nutr. Metab Care.* 6(6): 661–71.

Juraniæ Z, and Zizak Z 2005. Biological activities of berries: from antioxidant capacity to anti-cancer effects. *Biofactors* 23(4): 207–11.

Juroszek P, Lumpkin HM, Yang RY, Ledesma DR, and Ma CH 2009. Fruit quality and bioactive compounds with antioxidant activity of tomatoes grown on-farm: comparison of organic and conventional management systems. *J. Agric. Food Chem.* 57(4): 1188–94.

Korver O, 1997. 'Healthy' developments in the food industry. *Cancer Lett.* 114: 19–23.

Lerici C, and Giavedoni P 1994. Maillard reaction products. *In*: "Food Preservation by Combined Processes", Final report Flair C.A. Ed. ISBN 90–900–7303–5 EUR 15776 EN.

Lerici C, and Nicoli M 1996. Chemical and physico-chemical properties affecting the quality and stability of bakery products. *Adv. Food Sci.* (CMTL) 18: 229–233.

Lerici CR, 1998. Influence of modern technologies of processing, storage and distribution on food properties International seminar on nuclear war and planetary emergencies 23rd Session, (19–23 Aug. 1998), Erice, Italy.

Livny O, Reifen R, Levy I, Madar Z, Faulks R, Southon S, and Schwartz B 2003. Beta-carotene bioavailability from differently processed carrot meals in human ileostomy volunteers. *Eur. J. Nutr.* 42(6): 338–45.

Martí N, Mena P, Cánovas JA, Micol V, and Saura D 2009. Vitamin C and the role of citrus juices as functional food. *Nat. Prod. Commun.* 4(5): 677–700.

Nanditha B, and Prabhasankar P 2009. Antioxidants in bakery products: a review. *Crit. Rev. Food Sci. Nutr.* 49(1): 1–27.

Negi PS, and Roy SK 2003. Changes in beta-carotene and ascorbic acid content of fresh amaranth and fenugreek leaves during storage by low cost technique. *Plant Foods Hum. Nutr.* 58(3): 225–30.

Nemeth K, and Piskula MK 2007. Food content, processing, absorption and metabolism of onion flavonoids. *Crit. Rev. Food Sci. Nutr.* 47(4): 397–409.

Nicoli M, Anese M, Parpinel M, Franceschi S, and Lerici C 1997. Study on loss and/or formation of antioxidants in food during processing and storage. *Cancer Lett.* 114: 71–74.

Rodriguez-Amaya DB, 2003. Food carotenoids: analysis, composition and alterations during storage and processing of foods. *Forum Nutr.* 56: 35–7.

Worthington V, 2001. Nutritional quality of organic versus conventional fruits, vegetables, and grains. *J. Altern Complement Med.* 7(2): 161–73.

6

Review of Literature About Consumption of Fruits and Vegetables

Fruits and vegetables are the Mother Nature's gift to mankind, not just for adding flavor and color to our diets but for their richness in micronutrients, antioxidants and other nutraceuticals. Color of the fruits and vegetables has been mainly due to their flavonoids and carotenoids. However, some colorless fruits and vegetables are rich in vitamin C, other polyphenols like tannins which impart antioxidant action. Cruciferous vegetables like cabbage, broccoli and cauliflower are one of the dominant food crops worldwide which are widely considered to be healthy foods. They are high in vitamin C and soluble fibre and contain multiple nutrients with potent anti-cancer properties. Both diindolylmethane, sulforaphane, and many other sharp-tasting substances in these vegetables are synthesized glucosinolates.

STRATEGIES FOR IMPROVING FRUIT AND VEGETABLE INTAKES

Eating more fruits and vegetables and reducing dietary fat rank among the most important nutrition recommendations for health improvement. Telephone counseling is increasingly popular in delivering support for diet modification. Review was done by Vanwormer *et al.* (2006) to assess the effectiveness of telephone-based counseling on improving dietary fat, fruit, and vegetable consumption for adults through relevant randomized-controlled trials published during the past 5 years. Improvements were especially noticed among women with (or at high risk for developing) cancer. In some studies, telephone-based counseling was also associated with more improvement in blood lipid levels and weight. Telephone-based counseling was found to be a moderately effective intervention, but there are not enough studies yet to draw conclusions on points as how advantageous telephone-based counseling is, over traditional forms of dietary counseling. At present, telephone-based counseling may best be used as a complement to clinical care and a means to broaden the outreach of nutrition services (Vanwormer *et al.*, 2006).

Fruit and vegetable intake is generally inadequate among children due to preference for fast foods, sweets and snacks. A dietary counseling approach is needed to develop habit of eating fruits and vegetables. In a 12-week pilot intervention designed to encourage fruit and vegetable intake among 4th to 6th grade children (n=93) attending a YMCA summer camp, children participated in garden-based activities twice a week. Weekly educational activities included tests of fruit and vegetable tastes, preparing fruit and vegetable snacks, and family newsletters sent home to parents. Most children (97.8%) enjoyed taste-testing fruits and vegetables. Children also liked preparing fruit and vegetable snacks (93.4%), working in their garden (95.6%), and learning about fruits and vegetables (91.3%). Impact data suggested that this intervention led to an increase in the number of fruits and vegetables ever eaten ($p<0.001$), vegetable preferences ($p<0.001$), and fruit and vegetable asking behavior at home ($p<0.002$) and may help promote healthful eating behaviors among youth (Heim *et al.,* 2009; Michelle *et al.*, 2009). A High 5 for Preschool Kids (H5-KIDS) program tested the efficacy of a home based intervention to teach parents how to ensure a positive environment for their preschool child, and to examine whether changes in parent behavior were associated with improvements in child intake. When compared to control parents, H5-KIDS parents reported an increase in fruit-vegetable servings, knowledge and its availability within the home. H5-KIDS demonstrate the importance of participatory approaches in developing externally valid interventions, with the potential for dissemination across national parent education programs as a means for improving the intake of parents and young children (Haire-Joshu *et al.*, 2008).

Garden-based nutrition-education programs for youth are a promising strategy for improving preferences and increasing dietary intake of fruits and vegetables. Studies published between 1990 and 2007 were identified by Robinson-O'Brien *et al* (2009) through a library search of databases and examined the impact of garden-based nutrition education on fruit and/or vegetable intake, willingness to taste fruits and vegetables, preferences for fruits and vegetables, or other nutrition-related outcomes. Eleven studies were reviewed and included youth ranging in age from 5 to 15 years. Findings suggest that garden-based nutrition intervention programs may have the potential to promote increasing fruit and vegetable intake among youth and increased willingness to taste fruits and vegetables among younger children; however, empirical evidence in this area is relatively scanty (Robinson-O'Brien *et al.*, 2009). Sedentary lifestyles, along with diets low in fruits, vegetables, and complex carbohydrates and high in fat and total energy are common among youth. These unhealthy behaviors can contribute to an increase in childhood overweight, which is associated with type 2 diabetes, hypertension, and heart disease. Healthful dietary behaviors, such as eating a balanced and diverse diet may be addressed in garden-based programs for youth. The influence of a garden program, with a newly developed nutrition curriculum, on youth's eating and gardening behavior using the Theory of Planned Behavior was assessed in youth (age 8-15 years, n = 96). The model included the constructs of attitude, subjective norm, and perceived behavioral control (PBC). Since youth in the garden program consumed more fruit and vegetables at post-survey compared to pre-survey, it was concluded that garden programs may be a viable way to assist youth in making healthy lifestyle changes (Lautenschlager and Smith, 2007).

Use of focus group discussions was reported for web-based educational intervention to increase fruit and vegetable consumption on twelve groups (N=137, aged 21–65) from four geographically distinct health systems. Four groups were stratified by gender and eight by race (white and African American) and gender. Questions included their ideas about healthy eating, factors that encourage or serve as barriers to their consumption and features preferred for a web-based educational intervention. Results indicated motivators for consumption were being role models and health concerns. Barriers included lack of time, expense and availability (Rolnick *et al.*, 2009).

VEGETARIANISM AND FRUIT-VEGETABLE INTAKE

The consumption of fruits and vegetables is likely to be higher in vegetarians than the other groups. To investigate the relationships between vegetarianism, weight, dietary intake, and weight-control behaviors, a cross-sectional analysis was conducted a population-based study in Minnesota on both males and females (ages 15-23 years, n=2,516), through a mailed survey and food frequency questionnaire. Current vegetarians in the younger and older groups had healthier diets than nonvegetarians and were less likely to be overweight or obese (Robinson-O'Brien *et al.*, 2009).

To examine if counter parts adolescent vegetarians were more likely than nonvegetarian peers to meet the dietary recommendations of the Healthy People 2010 objectives and to examine differences in other nutrients between these 2 groups, 4746 adolescents from 31 middle and high schools in the Twin Cities area of Minnesota were surveyed. Participants were equally divided by sex. The mean age was 14.9 years with 34.3% were in junior high school and 65.7% in high school. The racial/ethnic distribution was 48.5% white, 19.0% African American, 19.2% Asian American, 5.8% Hispanic, 3.5% American Indian, and 3.9% others. Questions were asked on vegetarian status and whether eggs, dairy foods, chicken, fish were excluded. Dietary intake was assessed using the Youth and Adolescent Food Frequency Questionnaire. Vegetarian adolescents were found to be significantly more likely than non-vegetarian adolescents to meet the Healthy People 2010 objectives. This was particularly noteworthy for total fat (70% *vs* 48%), saturated fat (65% *vs* 39%), daily servings of vegetables (26% *vs* 14%), and 5 or more servings of fruits and vegetables (39% *vs* 28%). Vegetarians were also less likely to eat fast food, drink regular soda and fruit drinks. Vegetarians consumed less vitamin B12, more caffeine, and more iron. Study concluded that adolescent vegetarians showed a dietary pattern that is more likely than nonvegetarians to meet the Healthy People 2010 objectives (Perry *et al.*, 2002).

FACTORS INFLUENCING FRUIT AND VEGETABLE CONSUMPTION

The influencing factors of fruits and vegetables intakes such as personal factors, behavioral factors and socio-environmental factors have been studied. The study further aimed to identify correlates of home availability and taste preferences for fruits/vegetables, and to explore patterns of interaction between availability and taste preferences. The study population consisted of 3957 adolescents from 31 public middle and high schools in Minnesota. Structural equation modeling was used for model testing. The strongest correlates of fruit/vegetable intake were home availability of fruits/vegetables and taste preferences of fruits/

vegetables. The final model could explain 13% of the variance in fruit/vegetable intake, 45% of the variance in home availability, and 28% of the variance in taste preferences. Influencing factors of home availability included social support for healthy eating, family meal patterns, family food security, and socio-economic status. Correlates of taste preferences were health/nutrition attitudes and home availability of fruits/vegetables. Interaction effect of home availability of fruits/vegetables was low, intake patterns did not differ, regardless of taste preferences. In contrast, even when taste preferences for fruits/vegetables were low, if fruits/vegetables were available, intakes were increased. Interventions to increase fruit/vegetable intake in adolescents therefore need to target socio-environmental factors such as greater availability of fruits/vegetables (Neumark-Sztainer *et al.*, 2003).

LINKAGES OF FRUIT-VEGETABLE CONSUMPTION WITH CANCER

A factor analysis method was used to study associations between dietary patterns and colorectal cancer in middle-aged Americans. Diet was assessed among 293,615 men and 198,767 women in the National Institutes of Health-AARP Diet and Health Study. Principal components factor analysis identified 3 main dietary patterns: fruit and vegetables, diet foods, and red meat and potatoes pattern. State cancer registries identified 2151 incident cases of colorectal cancer in men and 959 in women between 1995 and 2000. Results suggested that dietary patterns a low frequency of meat and potato with consumption and frequent consumption of fruit and vegetables and fat-reduced foods are consistent with a decreased risk of colorectal cancer (Flood *et al.*, 2008 a). To determine the effects of dietary change on serum concentrations of insulin, glucose, IGF-I and IGFBP-3 a randomized clinical trial was conducted on 750 men and women (35 yr or more) without a history of who had at least one histologically confirmed colorectal adenoma After 4 years of follow-up, IGF-I concentration in the intervention group (n=248) declined by 8.86 ng/ml (initial men of 133 ng/ml (initial mean value of 139 ng/ml) in the non-intervention group (N=502). After 4 years, concentrations of IGFBP-3, insulin and glucose were not statistically different from values at baseline, and there were no differences in these serum measures between the intervention and control groups. A low-fat, high-fiber, high-fruit and –vegetable dietary intervention had minimal impact on serum concentrations of insulin, glucose, IGF-I and IGFBP-3 overall, but in lean subjects the intervention resulted in a significant reduction (Flood *et al.*, 2008 b).

Antioxidant nutrients present in fruits, vegetables and other foods are thought to prevent carcinogenesis and to influence immune status. A study conducted measuring consumption of fruits and vegetables for their influence on carcinogenesis and immune status has indicated greater intake of total fruits and vegetables (RR = 0.69; p = 0.011), yellow/orange (RR = 0.72; p = 0.015) and cruciferous (RR = 0.82; p = 0.017) vegetables, broccoli (RR = 0.72; p = 0.018) and apple juice/cider (RR = 0.65; p = 0.026) were associated with lower risk of cancer. These results supported a possible role of fruits and associated antioxidants from food sources, as protective factors against the development of NHL and follicular lymphoma in particular (Thompson *et al.*, 2010)

Cross-sectional associations between urinary albumin excretion and dietary patterns as well as intake of plant and animal foods were assessed in a study. A high consumption of low-fat dairy foods and a dietary pattern rich in whole grains, fruit, and low-fat dairy foods were both linked with lower urinary albumin-to-creatinine ratio. On the other hand, nondairy animal food intake was positively associated (Nettleton *et al.*, 2008).

Factors related to DNA damage and altered immunologic responses are also linked with the risk of non-Hodgkin lymphoma (NHL). To evaluate NHL risk with intakes of vegetables, fruit, and nutrients involved in antioxidant activities, a study was conducted on incident case subjects aged 20–74 y and age-sex matched control subjects 1321 case and 1057 control subjects were enrolled and dietary data were collected on a subset (466 cases and 391 controls). Carotenoid intakes were computed using updated USDA databases. NHL risk was found to be inversely associated with higher number of weekly servings of all vegetables. An influence of NHL subtype was observed with some food groups and nutrients. In particular, higher intakes of vegetables, lutein and zeaxanthin, and zinc reduced lower NHL risk (Kelemen *et al.*, 2006).

Although high vegetable intakes have been linked with a lower risk of colorectal cancer, this relation is not well established for the precursor lesions, adenomatous polyps. In a case-control design with adenomatous polyp cases (n = 564), colonoscopy-negative controls (polyp free at colonoscopy, n = 682), and community controls (n = 535), during 1991–1994 Minnesota Cancer Prevention Research Unit study investigated interrelationship between fruit and vegetable intake and first incident adenomatous polyps. Dietary intake was assessed using a food frequency questionnaire. For women, adenoma risk was half in the highest compared to lowest quintile of juice consumption (cases vs. colonoscopy-negative controls: odds ratio (OR) = 0.50, 95% confidence interval (CI): 0.27, 0.92; cases *vs.* community controls: OR = 0.56, 95% CI: 0.30, 1.06). The association was stronger for adenomas with moderate or severe types compared with mild dysplasia. Juice did not influence adenoma risk in men. The intakes of fruits, vegetables, total fruits and vegetables, green leafy vegetables, and several botanically and phytochemically defined subgroups were statistically not significant. Since higher vegetable intake has been associated with a lower risk of colorectal cancer, vegetables seem to have a stronger role in preventing the conversion of adenomas to carcinomas rather than in prevent the initial appearance of adenomas (Smith-Warner *et al.*, 2002).

The linkage between whole-grain intake and incident upper aerodigestive tract cancer in a cohort of 34,651 postmenopausal, women which were initially cancer-free was examined. The established risk factors for upper aerodigestive cancers, such as fruit and vegetable intake, smoking and alcohol intake were also included. During the 14-year follow-up period, 169 women developed cancer of the upper aerodigestive tract. For all cancers cases together, significant inverse associations were observed for the highest *vs* lowest tertile of whole grains (relative risk (RR) = 0.53, 95% confidence interval (CI) 0.34–0.81) and yellow/orange vegetables (RR = 0.58, 95% CI 0.39–0.87). In addition, those in the highest as compared to lowest tertile of fiber intake from whole grain were less likely to develop upper aerodigestive tract cancer (RR = 0.56, 95% CI 0.37–0.84) and fiber intake from refined grain was not significantly associated with upper aerodigestive tract cancer. Findings were more or less similar for oropharyngeal (n = 53), laryngeal (n = 21), nasopharyngeal/salivary (n = 18), esophageal (n = 21) and gastric (n = 56) cancers, though numbers of cases were very small for statistical testing within individual cancers. These findings confirmed previous observations that high intake of fruits and vegetables and that intake of whole grains with fiber derived from whole grains may reduce risk of upper aerodigestive tract cancers (Kasum *et al.*, 2002).

Case-control studies suggest a diet rich in fresh fruit and vegetables to protect from the risk of most common epithelial cancers which include that of digestive tract, and several other nondigestive neoplasms. However, selections in cohort studies have been generally weaker. To review the relation between frequency of consumption of vegetables and fruit, estimated intake of selected antioxidants and the risk of cancer at different sites were assessed. The relative risks (RR) of digestive tract neoplasms were lower in subjects having highest vegetable intake. A protective effect of vegetables has also been observed for hormone-related neoplasms. Fruit intake was related to lowered RR of cancers of the upper digestive tract, stomach and urinary tract. Considering the role of selected antioxidants, beta-carotene, vitamins C and E showed a significant inverse relation with oral and pharyngeal, esophageal and breast cancer risk. For colorectal cancer, the most consistent protective effects were provided by carotene, riboflavin and vitamin C, but inverse relations were observed also for calcium and vitamin D. Thus, fruit and vegetable intake in Mediterranean populations appears to provide protection against number of neoplasms (La Vecchia *et al.*, 2001).

FRUIT AND VEGETABLE INTAKE AND OTHER HEALTH PROBLEMS

Type 2 diabetics: Fruit and vegetable intake is found to be low for type 2 diabetics, which may be due to a perceived adverse effect on glycemic control. Cranberry juice consumption for type 2 diabetics represented an attractive option for increasing fruit intake and also affording positive health benefits as increase in plasma insulin and decrease in plasma glucose levels in one study. Cranberry juice may provide a favorable metabolic response and seem be useful for promoting increased fruit consumption for type 2 diabetics or others wishing to limit carbohydrate intake (Wilson *et al.*, 2008).

Deep vein thrombosis: There is no information on the role of dietary intake in the development of deep vein thrombosis or pulmonary embolus (venous thromboembolism (VTE)). Homocysteine, factor VIII, von Willebrand factor levels and risk factors for VTE are known to be influenced by dietary intake. A hypothesis that foods rich in B vitamins and omega-3 fatty acids are negatively associated and meat intake is positively associated with incidence of VTE was examined. In a prospective study conducted for over 12 years, 14,962 middle-aged adults participating in the atherosclerosis risk in communities study were followed up for incident of VTE. When all hospitalizations were identified, 196 VTEs were validated by chart review. A food frequency questionnaire assessed dietary intake at baseline and after 6 years. A diet with more plant foods and fish and less red and processed meat was associated with a reduced incidence of thromboembolism (Steffen *et al.*, 2007).

Cardiovascular disease: To examine whether dietary patterns can influence cardiovascular disease risk through effects on inflammation and endothelial activation, associations between dietary patterns and markers of inflammation and endothelial activation were assessed in 5089 nondiabetic participants in the Multi-Ethnic Study of Atherosclerosis. Four dietary patterns emerged using factor analysis. The fats and processed meats pattern (fats, oils, processed meats, fried potatoes, salty snacks, and desserts) was positively correlated with C-reactive protein (CRP) and homocysteine. The beans, tomatoes, and refined grains pattern (beans, tomatoes, refined grains, and high-fat dairy products) has positive impact on sICAM-1. But, the whole grains and fruit pattern (whole grains, fruit, nuts, and green leafy vegetables) was inversely associated with CRP, IL-6, homocysteine and sICAM-1 and the vegetables and fish pattern (fish and dark-yellow, cruciferous, and other vegetables) was inversely related to IL-6. These results confirm previous findings that empirically derived dietary patterns are associated with inflammation and show that these relations in an ethnically diverse population with unique dietary habits are similar to findings in more homogeneous populations (Nettleton *et al.*, 2006).

Rheumatoid arthritis: Relationship between antioxidant micronutrients and risk of rheumatoid arthritis in a cohort of older women was examined. After controlling for other risk factors, higher intakes of supplemental vitamin C and supplemental vitamin E were inversely associated with rheumatoid arthritis. There was no association with total carotenoids, alpha- or beta-carotene, lycopene, or lutein/ zeaxanthin, while there was an inverse association with beta-cryptoxanthin. Higher intakes of fruit and cruciferous vegetables also exhibited trends showing inverse associations with risk. When the antioxidants were modeled together, beta-cryptoxanthin and supplemental zinc were the only statistically significant predictors. Intake of some antioxidant micronutrients, viz beta-cryptoxanthin and supplemental zinc, and possibly diets high in fruits and cruciferous vegetables, seem to be protective against the development of rheumatoid arthritis (Cerhan *et al.*, 2003).

In general fruit and vegetable consumption can be increased through counseling of adolescents and children. Home availability and taste are significant influencing factors for intake of fruit and vegetables consumption of fruits and vegetables has a preventive effect rather than curative effect particularly on cancer.

REFERENCES

Cerhan JR, Saag KG, Merlino LA, *et al.* 2003. Antioxidant micronutrients and risk of rheumatoid arthritis in a cohort of older women. *Am. J. Epidemiol.* 157(4): 345–54.

Flood A, Mai V, Pfeiffer R, Kahle L, *et al.* 2008. The effects of a high-fruit and-vegetable, high-fiber, low-fat dietary intervention on serum concentrations of insulin, glucose, IGF-I, IGFBP-3 in serum glucose concentration. *Eur. J. Clin. Nutr.* 62(2): 186–96.

Flood A, Rastogi T, and Wirfält E, *et al.* 2008. Dietary patterns as identified by factor analysis and colorectal cancer in middle-aged Americans. *Am J. Clin. Nutr.* 88(1): 176–84.

Haire-Joshu D, Elliott MB, Caito NM, *et al.* 2008. High 5 for Kids: the impact of a home visiting program on fruit and vegetable intake of parents and their preschool children. *Prev. Med.* 47(1): 77–82.

Heims Stang J, and Ireland M 2009. A garden pilot project enhances fruit and vegetable consumption among children. *J. Am. Diet. Assoc.* 109(7): 1220-6.

Kasum CM, Jacobs DR Jr, Nicodemus K, and Folsom AR 2002. Dietary risk factors for upper aerodigestive tract cancers. *Int. J. Cancer.* 99(2): 267–72.

Kelemen LE, Cerhan JR, Lim U, *et al.* 2006. Vegetables, fruit, and antioxidant-related nutrients and risk of non-Hodgkin lymphoma: a National Cancer Institute-Surveillance, Epidemiology, and End Results population-based case-control study. *Am. J. Clin. Nutr.* 83(6): 1401–10.

La Vecchia C, Altieri A, and Tavani A 2001. Vegetables, fruit, antioxidants and cancer: a review of Italian studies. *Eur. J. Nutr.* 40(6): 261–7.

Lautenschlager L, and Smith C 2007. Understanding gardening and dietary habits among youth garden program participants using the Theory of Planned Behavior. *Appetite.* 49(1): 122–30.

Michelle M Ratcliffe, Kathleen A, *et al.* 2009. The Effects of School Garden Experiences on Middle School–Aged Students' Knowledge, Attitudes, and Behaviors Associated with Vegetable Consumption. *Health Promot Pract.* doi: 10.1177/1524839909349182.

Nettleton JA, Steffen LM, Mayer-Davis EJ, *et al.* 2006. Dietary patterns are associated with biochemical markers of inflammation and endothelial activation in the Multi-Ethnic Study of Atherosclerosis (MESA). *Am. J. Clin. Nutr.* 83(6): 1369–79.

Nettleton JA, Steffen LM, Palmas W, *et al.* 2008. Associations between microalbuminuria and animal foods, plant foods, and dietary patterns in the Multiethnic Study of Atherosclerosis. *Am J. Clin. Nutr.* 87(6): 1825–36.

Neumark-Sztainer D, Wall M, Perry C, and Story M 2003. Correlates of fruit and vegetable intake among adolescents. *Findings from Project EAT. Prev. Med.* 37(3): 198–208.

Perry CL, McGuire MT, Neumark-Sztainer D, and Story M 2002. Adolescent vegetarians: how well do their dietary patterns meet the healthy people 2010 objectives? *Arch. Pediatr. Adolesc. Med.* 156(5): 431–7.

Robinson-O'Brien R, Perry CL, Wall MM, Story M, and Neumark-Sztainer D 2009. Adolescent and young adult vegetarianism: better dietary intake and weight outcomes but increased risk of disordered eating behaviors. *J. Am. Diet. Assoc.* 109(4): 648–55.

Robinson-O'Brien R, Story M, and Heim S 2009. Impact of garden-based youth nutrition intervention programs: a review. *J. Am. Diet. Assoc.* 109(2): 273–80.

Rolnick SJ, Calvi J, Heimendinger J, *et al*. 2009. Patient Educ Couns. Focus groups inform a web-based program to increase fruit and vegetable intake. Patient Educational Counseling. 77(2): 314–8.

Smith-Warner SA, Elmer PJ, Fosdick L *et al*. 2002. Fruits, vegetables, and adenomatous polyps: the Minnesota Cancer Prevention Research Unit case-control study. *Am. J. Epidemiol.* 155(12): 1104–13.

Steffen LM, Folsom AR, Cushman M, *et al*. 2007. Greater fish, fruit, and vegetable intakes are related to lower incidence of venous thromboembolism: the Longitudinal Investigation of Thromboembolism Etiology. *Circulation*. 115(2): 188–95.

Thompson CA, Habermann TM, Wang AH, *et al*. 2010. Antioxidant intake from fruits, vegetables and other sources and risk of non-Hodgkin's lymphoma: the Iowa Women's Health Study). *Int. J. Cancer.* 126(4): 992–1003.

Vanwormer JJ, Boucher JL, and Pronk NP 2006. Telephone-based counseling improves dietary fat, fruit, and vegetable consumption: a best-evidence synthesis. *J. Am. Diet. Assoc.* 106(9): 1434–44.

Wilson T, Meyers SL, Singh AP *et al*. 2008. Favorable glycemic response of type 2 diabetics to low-calorie cranberry juice. *J. Food Sci.* 73(9): H241–5.

7

Development of Semi-Quantitative 'Antioxidant & Micronutrient Quality Index' (AQI and MQI)

INTRODUCTION

The science of nutrition has undergone a considerable evolution in last few decades. Energy and protein were in the focus for defining nutritious foods in earlier days. However, the research during last 2 decades has emerged with several new facets of micronutrients (vitamins and minerals) beyond their classical functions. Moreover, the so called anti-nutritional factors such as dietary fiber, polyphenols (tannins), enzyme inhibitors have now acquired the nutraceutical potentials. The antioxidant activity has got the most heightened revelation.

Recently modified food pyramid, emphasizes micronutrient quality of diet by giving importance to consumption of whole grains and a variety of fruits and vegetables (*mypyramid.gov*). Fruits and vegetables are rich sources of a variety of antioxidants and micronutrients (Tarwadi and Agte, 2006). In our study, popular fruits and vegetables such as guava, spinach, bitter gourd (*Momordica charantia*), yam, ginger and beetroot, and also less common ones like bael (*Aegle marmelos*), kokum (*Garcinia indica*) and mango-ginger (*Curcuma ameda*), showed potential *in vitro* to combat oxidative stress. (Annexure V) Further, we observed that there existed a large diversity in the contents of both antioxidants as well as individual micronutrients implicating thereby that all the fruits or vegetables are not equal in their antioxidant and micronutrient quality (Tarwadi and Agte, 2005). A need was therefore felt to develop a tool to assess the antioxidant (AQI) and micronutrient quality index (MQI) which can discriminate between fruits/vegetables rich in these healthy ingredients and poor sources. This tool can help in emphasizing specific fruits/vegetables rather than imparting comprehensive advice to consume more fruits and vegetables. The data collected for 4 vitamins, 4 trace metals and 4 antioxidant indices were used for this purpose (Annexure V).

APPROACH AND DEVELOPMENT OF A TOOL FOR AQI AND MQI

Initially a simple approach of arranging the individual members of each food group in increasing order and giving these an increasing rank was made as illustrated in Table 7.1. It was seen that chiku, banana, water melon were the low ranking fruits, while gooseberry, guava, tamrind, kokum were the top rankers. However, this approach was not found to be adequate to offer the rank which can correlate with observed values. For example, if banana is the poorest having rank 23 and gooseberry is the rich fruit having rank 93, it would not give any idea as to what is the equivalence of one gooseberry in terms of bananas. Thus the ideal tool needs to have the point system and instead of ranks, individual food needs to be given scores based on point system.

As a next step, each of the values for antioxidant indices were so modified with constant multiplier that highest value would get the rank of 10 and all the values would lie between 0 to 10. The values of AQI were then rounded to get a single digit number as shown in Table 7.2. This approach could give ranks, their relative gradation due to multiplication with constant number to all the values and uniformity of numbers. One weak point in this approach was that the MQI ranks, though showing relative potentials with respect to each other, did not give any idea about how good any food is to fulfill the recommended dietary allowance (RDA). (Tables 7.3–7.10)

For assessing the quality of micronutrients therefore a new index of computing RDI units/100 g was attempted and the data from all the 4 assessed food groups *viz.* green leafy vegetables (GLV), fruits, fruit vegetables and root vegetables were ranked based on the RDA values for each of the assessed micronutrient.

Tables 7.11 and 7.12 show MQI based on the amounts of RDA met for vitamins and trace minerals by fruits and vegetables. As seen in Table 7.11, big amla, small amla (Raiamla) followed by guava showed highest ranks, meaning thereby that 100 g of these fruits can give of 8.7, 8.2 and 3.8% of RDA. On the other hand, Zyziphus with rank 0.06 can meet RDA by only 6%. Table 7.12 gives similar ranks for trace metals.

Table 7.1: Ranking of fruits based on antioxidant indices

FRUITS	*Values/100g*					*Ranks*				
	Energy Kcals	*ITBARS mM Vitamin E*	*SOSA mM tannic acid*	*FICA mM EDTA*	*Poly-phenols mg*	*ITBARS*	*SOSA*	*FICA*	*Poly-phenols*	*Pooled*
Apple	59	0.61	25.48	56.74	142.1	23	13	30	22	88
Banana big	116	0.59	14.65	9.3	50	21	5	1	10	37
Banana small	–	0.23	2.7	9.98	63.8	7	1	2	13	23
Bel fruit	137	0.19	77.19	62.44	104.4	5	32	32	19	88
Big amla	58	0.6	18.3	61.67	1324	22	9	31	31	93
Carrisa	–	0.56	19.66	18.68	177.6	20	11	7	25	63
Cashew fruit	51	0.67	54.16	49.11	49.31	27	29	27	8	91
Chiku	98	0.24	11.67	15.11	23.9	9	2	4	1	16
Dalimb	65	0.61	13.1	29.9	200	24	4	11	28	67
Guava	51	0.97	34.35	47.81	97.8	32	19	25	17	93
Kokum	–	0.81	42.93	39.68	259.6	31	24	20	30	105
Lemon	57	0.54	43.3	41.29	32.6	19	25	22	3	69
Mango alphanso	74	0.28	19.13	31.12	39.8	10	10	13	6	39
Musk melon	17	0.13	14.89	20.42	124.7	2	6	8	20	36
Pear	52	0.64	40.41	11.64	24.65	26	23	3	2	54
Orange	48	0.3	16.32	33.16	77.5	13	8	14	14	49
Papaya	32	0.3	30.32	40.68	86.3	14	17	21	16	68
Pineapple	46	0.28	28.74	46.9	101.5	11	16	24	18	69
Raiamla	–	0.8	47.8	30.55	1356	30	28	12	32	102

Table 7.1: (*Contd...*)

Table 7.1: (*Contd...*)

FRUITS	*Values/100g*					*Ranks*				
	Energy Kcals	*ITBARS mM Vitamin E*	*SOSA mM tannic acid*	*FICA mM EDTA*	*Poly-phenols mg*	*ITBARS*	*SOSA*	*FICA*	*Poly-phenols*	*Pooled*
Ramphal	70	0.49	27.9	33.74	39.15	17	14	15	5	51
Rose apple	39	0.127	44.05	48.8	221.1	1	26	26	29	82
Seethaphal	104	0.67	34	45.68	53.6	28	18	23	11	80
Strawberry	44	0.36	22.68	18.64	54.4	16	12	6	12	46
Sweet lime	43	0.23	45.92	28.91	40.6	8	27	10	7	52
Tamarind red	283	0.53	58.33	52.85	143.5	18	30	28	23	99
Tamarind white	–	0.29	35.37	38.76	81.9	12	20	18	15	65
Water chestnut	–	0.74	60.88	53.78	188.1	29	31	29	26	115
Water melon	16	0.17	12.66	16.45	141.4	4	3	5	21	33
Wood apple	134	0.34	28.54	20.67	167.5	15	15	9	24	63
Ziziphus big	74	0.22	35.74	35.05	195.8	6	21	17	27	71
Ziziphus small	–	0.61	16.24	33.76	49.6	25	7	16	9	57
Ziziphus yellow	–	0.16	35.75	39.24	37.8	3	22	19	4	48

Table 7.2: Modified ranking of fruits based on antioxidant indices

	Values					*Ranks*			
FRUITS	***Energy***	***ITBARS***	***SOSA***	***FICA***	***Polyphenols***	***ITBARS***	***SOSA***	***FICA***	***Polyphenols***
Apple	59	0.61	25.48	56.74	142.1	6	3	6	1
Banana big	116	0.59	14.65	9.3	50	6	1	1	1
Banana small	–	0.23	2.7	9.98	63.8	2	0	1	1
Bel fruit	137	0.19	77.19	62.44	104.4	2	8	6	1
Big amla	58	0.6	18.3	61.67	1324	6	2	6	13
Carrisa	–	0.56	19.66	18.68	177.6	6	2	2	2
Cashew fruit	51	0.67	54.16	49.11	49.31	7	5	5	0
Chiku	98	0.24	11.67	15.11	23.9	2	1	2	0
Dalimb	65	0.61	13.1	29.9	200	6	1	3	2
Guava	51	0.97	34.35	47.81	97.8	10	3	5	1
Kokum	–	0.81	42.93	39.68	259.6	8	4	4	3
Lemon	57	0.54	43.3	41.29	32.6	5	4	4	0
Mango alphanso	74	0.28	19.13	31.12	39.8	3	2	3	0
Musk melon	17	0.13	14.89	20.42	124.7	1	1	2	1
Naspatti	52	0.64	40.41	11.64	24.65	6	4	1	0
Orange	48	0.3	16.32	33.16	77.5	3	2	3	1
Papaya	32	0.3	30.32	40.68	86.3	3	3	4	1
Pineapple	46	0.28	28.74	46.9	101.5	3	3	5	1
Raiamla	–	0.8	47.8	30.55	1356	8	5	3	14
Ramphal	70	0.49	27.9	33.74	39.15	5	3	3	0
Rose apple	39	0.127	44.05	48.8	221.1	1	4	5	2

Table 7.2: (*Contd...*)

Table 7.2: (*Contd...*)

	Values					*Ranks*			
FRUITS	***Energy***	***ITBARS***	***SOSA***	***FICA***	***Polyphenols***	***ITBARS***	***SOSA***	***FICA***	***Polyphenols***
Seethaphal	104	0.67	34	45.68	53.6	7	3	5	1
Strawberry	44	0.36	22.68	18.64	54.4	4	2	2	1
Sweet lime	43	0.23	45.92	28.91	40.6	2	5	3	0
Tamarind red	283	0.53	58.33	52.85	143.5	5	6	5	1
Tamarind white	–	0.29	35.37	38.76	81.9	3	4	4	1
Water chestnut	–	0.74	60.88	53.78	188.1	7	6	5	2
Water melon	16	0.17	12.66	16.45	141.4	2	1	2	1
Wood apple	134	0.34	28.54	20.67	167.5	3	3	2	2
Ziziphus big	74	0.22	35.74	35.05	195.8	2	4	4	2
Ziziphus small	–	0.61	16.24	33.76	49.6	6	2	3	0
Ziziphus yellow	–	0.16	35.75	39.24	37.8	2	4	4	0
Mean	73.7	0.45	31.661	35.08	179.69	–	–	–	–
s.d.	55.5	0.23	16.83	15.21	311.14	–	–	–	–
Median	57.5	0.42	29.53	34.41	92.05	–	–	–	–

Table 7.3: Amount of RDA for vitamins met from fruits and their ranks

FRUITS	*Vit C*	*β carotene*	*Riboflavin*	*Thiamine*	*Rank*
Mango alphanso	0.30	500.00	0.07	0.02	500.39
Guava	3.70	26.67	0.02	0.01	30.39
Wood apple	1.10	26.67	0.02	0.02	27.80
Rose apple	0.30	26.67	0.02	0.02	27.01
Bullock's heart	0.08	26.67	0.01	0.02	26.77
Strawberry	1.03	23.33	0.01	0.03	24.40
Cashew fruit	0.25	23.33	0.02	0.03	23.62
Sapota	0.10	22.50	0.01	0.01	22.62
Papaya	0.40	20.00	0.01	0.01	20.42
Sweet lime	1.03	16.67	0.02	0.01	17.72
Kokum fruit	0.50	16.67	0.02	0.01	17.20
Big gooseberry	8.63	6.67	0.02	0.03	15.34
Naspatti	0.25	15.00	0.01	0.01	15.27
Raigooseberry	8.13	6.67	0.01	0.01	14.82
Pineapple	0.40	13.33	0.11	0.03	13.88
Orange	0.83	10.00	0.03	0.03	10.88
Carrisa	0.58	10.00	0.01	0.02	10.61
Tamarind red	0.30	10.00	0.01	0.01	10.32
Custard apple	0.25	10.00	0.02	0.02	10.29
Ziziphus yellow	0.20	10.00	0.01	0.01	10.22
Tamarind white	0.20	10.00	0.01	0.01	10.22
Water chestnut	0.15	10.00	0.01	0.01	10.17
Banana small	0.10	10.00	0.01	0.02	10.12
Ziziphus big	0.03	10.00	0.01	0.01	10.05
Pomegranate	0.40	6.67	0.01	0.01	7.09
Banana big	0.10	6.67	0.01	0.02	6.79
Ziziphus small	0.08	6.67	0.01	0.01	6.76
Lemon	0.70	3.33	0.01	0.01	4.06
Bel fruit	0.30	3.33	0.01	0.03	3.67
Apple	0.13	3.33	0.01	0.02	3.49
Water melon	0.08	3.33	0.01	0.01	3.42
Musk melon	0.05	3.33	0.01	0.01	3.40

Table 7.4: Amount of RDA for trace metals met from fruits and their ranks

FRUITS	*Zinc*	*Iron*	*Manganese*	*Selenium*	*Copper*	*Rank*
Bel fruit	0.01	0.02	0.02	2.20	0.02	2.26
Ziziphus small	0.02	0.00	0.05	1.64	0.02	1.73
Sweet lime	0.02	0.01	0.17	1.40	0.02	1.61
Pomegranate	0.00	0.01	0.02	1.28	0.02	1.33
Pear	0.00	0.01	0.01	1.28	0.01	1.31
Small gooseberry	0.00	0.00	0.04	1.24	0.01	1.29
Banana big	0.01	0.02	0.01	1.20	0.01	1.24
Musk melon	0.01	0.01	0.03	1.16	0.02	1.23
Apple	0.00	0.00	0.01	1.00	0.01	1.03
Banana small	0.01	0.02	0.02	0.92	0.01	0.98
Pineapple	0.00	0.00	0.02	0.88	0.01	0.91
Papaya	0.01	0.01	0.03	0.80	0.03	0.87
Big gooseberry	0.00	0.01	0.03	0.80	0.02	0.86
Ramphal	0.00	0.01	0.04	0.68	0.01	0.74
Tamarind red	0.02	0.01	0.12	0.48	0.02	0.65
Orange	0.00	0.01	0.01	0.56	0.02	0.60
Ziziphus yellow	0.01	0.05	0.08	0.40	0.01	0.55
Tamarind white	0.01	0.01	0.03	0.44	0.03	0.52
Carrisa	0.01	0.01	0.04	0.44	0.01	0.50
Lemon	0.05	0.00	0.04	0.36	0.02	0.48
Water melon	0.00	0.00	0.01	0.40	0.02	0.43
Cashew fruit	0.01	0.01	0.03	0.36	0.01	0.41
Mango alphanso	0.00	0.00	0.02	0.32	0.01	0.35
Strawberry	0.01	0.01	0.03	0.28	0.02	0.34
Guava	0.00	0.00	0.01	0.28	0.01	0.31
Ziziphus big	0.00	0.00	0.04	0.20	0.01	0.25
Water chestnut	0.00	0.00	0.02	0.20	0.01	0.23
Rose apple	0.00	0.00	0.02	0.20	0.01	0.23
Wood apple	0.00	0.00	0.02	0.20	0.00	0.22
Sapota	0.00	0.00	0.03	0.12	0.01	0.17
Custard apple	0.00	0.00	0.01	0.08	0.01	0.10
Kokum fruit	0.00	0.00	0.01	0.04	0.03	0.09

Table 7.5: Amount of RDA for vitamins met from GLV and their ranks

GLV	*Vit C*	*β carotene*	*Riboflavin*	*Thiamine*	*Rank*
Colocasia black	1.06	2946.67	0.07	0.03	2947.83
Colocasia green	0.35	2365.83	0.10	0.04	2366.33
Curry leaves	0.06	2170.00	0.07	0.07	2170.20
Coriander	2.23	2110.00	0.04	0.03	2112.30
Drumstick	3.50	2060.00	0.02	0.02	2063.54
Shepu	0.40	2026.67	0.07	0.02	2027.15
Amaranthus red	1.85	1985.00	0.06	0.06	1986.97
Raddish	1.74	1936.67	0.08	0.03	1938.51
Amaranthus green	1.40	1726.67	0.08	0.03	1728.18
Spinach	0.50	1403.33	0.09	0.03	1403.95
Safflower	0.48	1376.67	0.08	0.04	1377.27
Cauliflower	0.17	1296.67	0.09	0.04	1296.97
Chakvat	0.45	1293.33	0.09	0.07	1293.93
Ambat chuka	0.20	883.33	0.07	0.04	883.65
Omum	0.53	875.83	0.06	0.04	876.46
Fenugreek	0.64	836.67	0.06	0.06	837.43
Gogu	0.37	557.50	0.08	0.03	557.98
Beet greens	0.41	427.50	0.08	0.03	428.02
Lettuce	0.12	393.33	0.07	0.03	393.55
Onion stalks	0.32	380.83	0.09	0.05	381.30
Knol-Khol greens	0.57	380.00	0.09	0.03	380.68
Mint	0.04	374.58	0.06	0.03	374.71
Patardi	0.26	340.83	0.10	0.04	341.23
Carrot greens	0.51	315.83	0.11	0.05	316.50
Amaranthus vir	0.70	296.67	0.09	0.03	297.49
Cabbage	0.16	203.33	0.07	0.02	203.58
Keni	0.32	134.17	0.07	0.05	134.61
Tamrind	0.03	77.08	0.09	0.07	77.27
Fetid cassia	1.26	10.00	0.07	0.07	11.40

Table 7.6: Amount of RDA for trace metals met from GLV and their ranks

GLV	*Zinc*	*Copper*	*Iron*	*Manganese*	*Selenium*	*Rank*
Amaranthus red	0.01	0.02	0.76	0.84	0.09	1.71
Chakvat	0.00	0.01	1.00	0.52	0.16	1.70
Raddish	0.01	0.05	0.44	0.88	0.01	1.38
Onion greens	0.01	0.02	0.84	0.48	0.01	1.36
Omum	0.01	0.01	0.24	0.76	0.06	1.08
Cauliflower	0.01	0.01	0.08	0.80	0.14	1.03
Safflower	0.01	0.02	0.17	0.68	0.14	1.01
Colocasia black	0.01	0.04	0.28	0.56	0.09	0.98
Fetid cassia	0.01	0.01	0.46	0.40	0.09	0.97
Curry leaves	0.01	0.01	0.19	0.64	0.04	0.89
Fenugreek	0.01	0.01	0.05	0.76	0.06	0.89
Shepu	0.01	0.02	0.39	0.40	0.07	0.89
Colocasia green	0.00	0.02	0.29	0.48	0.09	0.89
Drumstick	0.01	0.01	0.30	0.40	0.09	0.81
Coriander	0.00	0.01	0.06	0.56	0.17	0.80
Ambat chuka	0.01	0.02	0.21	0.40	0.14	0.78
Carrot greens	0.01	0.04	0.08	0.60	0.04	0.76
Tamrind	0.00	0.02	0.08	0.56	0.06	0.72
Patardi	0.01	0.01	0.09	0.56	0.03	0.71
Amaranthus green	0.01	0.03	0.08	0.44	0.09	0.65
Lettuce	0.00	0.01	0.11	0.38	0.14	0.64
Spinach	0.01	0.02	0.03	0.44	0.09	0.59
Gogu	0.01	0.02	0.08	0.48	0.00	0.58
Knol-Khol greens	0.00	0.00	0.04	0.40	0.05	0.49
Keni	0.00	0.01	0.04	0.36	0.08	0.49
Cabbage	0.00	0.00	0.03	0.40	0.04	0.47
Beet greens	0.01	0.04	0.06	0.20	0.03	0.34
Mint	0.01	0.00	0.02	0.20	0.01	0.23

Table 7.7: Amount of RDA for vitamins met from fruit vegetables and their ranks

Fruit-Vegetables	*Vit C*	*β carotene*	*Riboflavin*	*Thiamine*	*Rank*
Capsicum	0.33	76.25	0.01	0.02	76.61
Coccinea	0.10	29.17	0.01	0.02	29.30
Brinjal purple	0.03	24.17	0.03	0.02	24.24
Bitter gourd	0.29	21.25	0.02	0.02	21.58
Brinjal green large	0.11	20.83	0.03	0.02	20.99
Tomato green	0.23	20.42	0.01	0.02	20.67
Cauliflower	0.09	18.75	0.02	0.02	18.88
Tomato red	0.19	13.75	0.01	0.03	13.98
Ladies finger	0.10	12.50	0.02	0.03	12.66
Red pumpkin	0.06	10.42	0.01	0.04	10.54
Brinjal green small	0.05	9.58	0.02	0.01	9.67
Bottle gourd	0.05	8.33	0.01	0.02	8.41
Ridge gourd	0.11	4.58	0.01	0.03	4.74

Table 7.8: Amount of RDA for trace metals met from fruit vegetables and their ranks

Fruit-Vegetables	*Zinc*	*Copper*	*Iron*	*Manganese*	*Selenium*	*Rank*
Brinjal green large	0.02	0.03	0.08	0.14	1.46	1.73
Ridge gourd	0.01	0.05	0.10	0.29	1.20	1.66
Tomato red	0.01	0.02	0.09	0.27	0.90	1.29
Tomato green	0.03	0.01	0.04	0.27	0.93	1.28
Red pumpkin	0.02	0.02	0.06	0.06	1.07	1.23
Brinjal purp.	0.02	0.05	0.02	0.02	0.94	1.05
Ladies finger	0.01	0.01	0.08	0.12	0.75	0.98
Brinjal green small	0.02	0.04	0.04	0.08	0.66	0.83
Bitter gourd	0.02	0.01	0.05	0.31	0.36	0.76
Bottle gourd	0.01	0.01	0.02	0.04	0.57	0.65
Cauliflower	0.02	0.01	0.07	0.09	0.25	0.45
Coccinea	0.02	0.02	0.06	0.05	0.18	0.32
Capsicum	0.01	0.01	0.04	0.02	0.18	0.25

Table 7.9: Amount of RDA for vitamins met from root vegetables and their ranks

Root vegetables	*Vit C*	*β carotene*	*Riboflavin*	*Thiamine*	*Rank*
Ginger	0.11	39.17	0.02	0.02	39.33
Garlic	0.06	32.50	0.01	0.02	32.59
Onion red	0.03	31.67	0.02	0.02	31.74
Onion white	0.24	28.33	0.02	0.02	28.61
Potato	0.25	26.25	0.01	0.02	26.53
Sweet potato	0.04	20.42	0.01	0.02	20.48
Raddish white	0.02	18.75	0.01	0.02	18.80
Raddish red	0.01	16.67	0.01	0.03	16.72
Colocasia	0.11	13.75	0.01	0.02	13.88
Yam	0.06	13.75	0.01	0.02	13.85
Turnip	0.06	11.67	0.02	0.02	11.77
Beetroot	0.04	7.92	0.01	0.01	7.99
Mango ginger white	0.21	7.08	0.02	0.02	7.33
Mango ginger yellow	0.21	5.83	0.02	0.01	6.08
Carrot	0.06	515.42	0.01	0.02	515.52

Table 7.10: Amount of RDA for trace metals met from root vegetables and their ranks

Root vegetables	*Zinc*	*Copper*	*Iron*	*Manganese*	*Selenium*	*Rank*
Mango ginger yellow	0.03	0.12	0.10	0.62	4.50	5.37
Turnip	0.01	0.07	0.09	0.67	3.10	3.94
Onion red	0.03	0.05	0.04	0.47	3.00	3.58
Ginger	0.04	0.12	0.02	0.85	2.10	3.14
Raddish red	0.01	0.12	0.09	0.58	2.30	3.11
Garlic	0.02	0.06	0.04	0.29	2.10	2.51
Carrot	0.03	0.10	0.05	0.49	1.50	2.16
Sweet potato	0.04	0.25	0.01	0.42	1.30	2.02
Onion white	0.01	0.06	0.03	0.38	1.30	1.78
Potato	0.01	0.05	0.01	0.40	1.30	1.77
Beetroot	0.01	0.02	0.07	0.29	1.30	1.69
Raddish white	0.01	0.09	0.02	0.04	1.40	1.55
Mango ginger white	0.07	0.06	0.01	0.47	0.60	1.21
Colocasia	0.03	0.10	0.01	0.20	0.50	0.83
Yam	0.03	0.12	0.01	0.25	0.20	0.61

Table 7.11: Ranks based on relative contribution with respect to RDA

Fruits	*Vitamin C*	*Beta carotene*	*Riboflavin*	*Thiamine*	*Pooled Rank*
Big amla	8.63	0.01	0.02	0.03	8.68
Rai amla	8.13	0.01	0.01	0.01	8.16
Guava	3.70	0.03	0.02	0.01	3.75
Wood apple	1.10	0.03	0.02	0.02	1.16
Strawberry	1.03	0.02	0.01	0.03	1.09
Sweet lime	1.03	0.02	0.02	0.01	1.07
Orange	0.83	0.01	0.03	0.03	0.89
Mango alphanso	0.30	0.50	0.07	0.02	0.89
Lemon	0.70	0.00	0.01	0.01	0.73
Carrisa	0.58	0.01	0.01	0.02	0.62
Pineapple	0.40	0.01	0.11	0.03	0.56
Kokum	0.50	0.02	0.02	0.01	0.55
Papaya	0.40	0.02	0.01	0.01	0.44
Dalimb	0.40	0.01	0.01	0.01	0.43
Rose apple	0.30	0.03	0.02	0.02	0.37
Bel fruit	0.30	0.00	0.01	0.03	0.34
Tamarind red	0.30	0.01	0.01	0.01	0.33
Cashew fruit	0.25	0.02	0.02	0.03	0.31
Seethaphal	0.25	0.01	0.02	0.02	0.30
Pear	0.25	0.02	0.01	0.01	0.28
Ziziphus yellow	0.20	0.01	0.01	0.01	0.23
Tamarind white	0.20	0.01	0.01	0.01	0.23
Water chestnut	0.15	0.01	0.01	0.01	0.18
Apple	0.13	0.00	0.01	0.02	0.16
Sapota	0.10	0.02	0.01	0.01	0.14
Banana small	0.10	0.01	0.01	0.02	0.13
Ramphal	0.08	0.03	0.01	0.02	0.13
Banana big	0.10	0.01	0.01	0.02	0.13
Ziziphus small	0.08	0.01	0.01	0.01	0.10
Water melon	0.08	0.00	0.01	0.01	0.09
Musk melon	0.05	0.00	0.01	0.01	0.07
Ziziphus big	0.03	0.01	0.01	0.01	0.06

Table 7.12: Ranks based on relative contribution of minerals with respect to RDA

Fruits	*Zinc*	*Iron*	*Manganese*	*Copper*	*Pooled Rank*
Sweet lime	0.023	0.008	0.167	0.016	0.215
Tamarind red	0.020	0.012	0.116	0.024	0.172
Ziziphus yellow	0.006	0.053	0.080	0.011	0.150
Lemon	0.049	0.002	0.044	0.022	0.117
Ziziphus sml	0.018	0.003	0.051	0.016	0.087
Tamarind white	0.010	0.013	0.025	0.029	0.077
Papaya	0.006	0.012	0.029	0.027	0.074
Musk melon	0.005	0.005	0.035	0.024	0.069
Big amla	0.003	0.014	0.029	0.018	0.064
Bel fruit	0.007	0.023	0.017	0.016	0.063
Carrisa	0.007	0.010	0.036	0.009	0.063
Ramphal	0.004	0.009	0.044	0.005	0.063
Banana small	0.007	0.016	0.022	0.015	0.059
Strawberry	0.005	0.006	0.025	0.022	0.059
Cashew fruit	0.005	0.007	0.028	0.013	0.053
Dalimb	0.004	0.007	0.017	0.024	0.052
Raiamla	0.003	0.003	0.036	0.009	0.052
Ziziphus big	0.004	0.002	0.036	0.009	0.051
Chikku	0.004	0.004	0.033	0.009	0.051
Kokum	0.004	0.005	0.011	0.029	0.048
Banana big	0.005	0.020	0.011	0.007	0.044
Orange	0.001	0.007	0.005	0.022	0.035
Water chestnut	0.004	0.001	0.022	0.007	0.034
Mango alphanso	0.003	0.003	0.018	0.007	0.031
Water melon	0.004	0.001	0.007	0.018	0.030
Naspatti	0.004	0.006	0.015	0.005	0.030
Pineapple	0.002	0.005	0.017	0.005	0.029
Rose apple	0.003	0.004	0.016	0.005	0.029
Apple	0.003	0.004	0.009	0.011	0.027
Guava	0.004	0.001	0.015	0.005	0.026
Seethaphal	0.003	0.002	0.010	0.007	0.023
Wood apple	0.003	0.001	0.015	0.004	0.022

In this case, sweet lime, tamarind and ziziphus yellow had highest ranks while wood apple and custard apple were at the bottom. As seen in Tables 7.13 and 7.14, for GLVs, drumstick, coriander had highest rank for vitamin-MQI and amarathus red and chakvat for trace metal-MQI. Among the fruit and root vegetables top rankers for vitamin-MQI were

Table 7.13: Ranks based on relative contribution of vitamins with respect to RDA

GLV	*Vit C*	*Beta carotene*	*Riboflavin*	*Thiamine*	*Pooled Rank*
Drumstick	3.50	2.06	0.02	0.02	5.60
Coriander	2.23	2.11	0.04	0.03	4.41
Colocasia black	1.06	2.95	0.07	0.03	4.11
Amaranthus red	1.85	1.99	0.06	0.06	3.96
Raddish	1.74	1.94	0.08	0.03	3.78
Amaranthus green	1.40	1.73	0.08	0.03	3.24
Colocasia green	0.35	2.37	0.10	0.04	2.86
Shepu	0.40	2.03	0.07	0.02	2.51
Curry leaves	0.06	2.17	0.07	0.07	2.37
Spinach	0.50	1.40	0.09	0.03	2.02
Safflower	0.48	1.38	0.08	0.04	1.98
Chakvat	0.45	1.29	0.09	0.07	1.89
Fetid cassia	1.26	0.27	0.07	0.07	1.67
Cauliflower	0.17	1.30	0.09	0.04	1.60
Fenugreek	0.64	0.84	0.06	0.06	1.60
Omum	0.53	0.88	0.06	0.04	1.50
Ambat chuka	0.20	0.88	0.07	0.04	1.20
Amaranthus vir	0.70	0.30	0.09	0.03	1.12
Knol-Khol greens	0.57	0.38	0.09	0.03	1.06
Gogu	0.37	0.56	0.08	0.03	1.04
Carrot greens	0.51	0.32	0.11	0.05	0.98
Beet greens	0.41	0.43	0.08	0.03	0.95
Onion stalks	0.32	0.38	0.09	0.05	0.84
Patardi	0.26	0.34	0.10	0.04	0.74
Lettuce	0.12	0.39	0.07	0.03	0.61
Keni	0.32	0.13	0.07	0.05	0.58
Mint	0.04	0.37	0.06	0.03	0.50
Cabbage	0.16	0.20	0.07	0.02	0.45
Tamarind	0.03	0.10	0.09	0.07	0.29

capsicum, bitter gourd, carrot and for trace metal-MQI were brinjal, ridge gourd and mango ginger and turnip (Tables 7.15 and 7.16).

Lastly, an attempt was made to pool all the food groups and ranks for both vitamins and trace metals. The best performing foods came out to be two types of amla and guava which could be due to their high contents of vitamin C relative to it's RDA (Tables 7.17 and 7.18) Sample calculation is shown in Table 7.19. Review of literature on development of quality index has been given in Annexure VII.

Table 7.14: Ranks based on relative contribution with respect to RDA

GLV	*Zinc*	*Copper*	*Iron*	*Manganese*	*Selenium*	*Pooled Rank*
Amaranthus red	0.01	0.02	0.76	0.84	0.09	1.71
Chakvat	0.00	0.01	1.00	0.52	0.16	1.70
Raddish	0.01	0.05	0.44	0.88	0.01	1.38
Onion greens	0.01	0.02	0.84	0.48	0.01	1.36
Omum	0.01	0.01	0.24	0.76	0.06	1.08
Cauliflower	0.01	0.01	0.08	0.80	0.14	1.03
Safflower	0.01	0.02	0.17	0.68	0.14	1.01
Colocasia black	0.01	0.04	0.28	0.56	0.09	0.98
Fetid cassia	0.01	0.01	0.46	0.40	0.09	0.97
Curry leaves	0.01	0.01	0.19	0.64	0.04	0.89
Fenugreek	0.01	0.01	0.05	0.76	0.06	0.89
Shepu	0.01	0.02	0.39	0.40	0.07	0.89
Colocasia green	0.00	0.02	0.29	0.48	0.09	0.89
Drumstick	0.01	0.01	0.30	0.40	0.09	0.81
Coriander	0.00	0.01	0.06	0.56	0.17	0.80
Ambat chuka	0.01	0.02	0.21	0.40	0.14	0.78
Carrot greens	0.01	0.04	0.08	0.60	0.04	0.76
Tamrind	0.00	0.02	0.08	0.56	0.06	0.72
Patardi	0.01	0.01	0.09	0.56	0.03	0.71
Amaranthus green	0.01	0.03	0.08	0.44	0.09	0.65
Lettuce	0.00	0.01	0.11	0.38	0.14	0.64
Spinach	0.01	0.02	0.03	0.44	0.09	0.59
Gogu	0.01	0.02	0.08	0.48	0.00	0.58
Knol-Khol greens	0.00	0.00	0.04	0.40	0.05	0.49
Keni	0.00	0.01	0.04	0.36	0.08	0.49
Cabbage	0.00	0.00	0.03	0.40	0.04	0.47
Beet greens	0.01	0.04	0.06	0.20	0.03	0.34
Mint	0.01	0.00	0.02	0.20	0.01	0.23

Table 7.15: Ranks based on relative contribution with respect to RDA

Fruit vegetables	*Vit C*	*β carotene*	*Riboflavin*	*Thiamine*	*Rank*
Capsicum	0.33	0.08	0.01	0.02	0.43
Bitter gourd	0.29	0.02	0.02	0.02	0.35
Tomato green	0.23	0.02	0.01	0.02	0.27
Tomato red	0.19	0.01	0.01	0.03	0.24
Brinjal green large	0.11	0.02	0.03	0.02	0.17
Ladies finger	0.10	0.01	0.02	0.03	0.17
Ridge gourd	0.11	0.00	0.01	0.03	0.16
Coccinea	0.10	0.03	0.01	0.02	0.16
Cauliflower	0.09	0.02	0.02	0.02	0.14
Red pumpkin	0.06	0.01	0.01	0.04	0.13
Brinjal purple	0.03	0.02	0.03	0.02	0.10
Brinjal green small	0.05	0.01	0.02	0.01	0.09
Bottle gourd	0.05	0.01	0.01	0.02	0.09
Carrot	0.06	0.52	0.01	0.02	0.62
Mango ginger yellow	0.25	0.03	0.01	0.02	0.31
Mango ginger white	0.24	0.03	0.02	0.02	0.30
Raddish white	0.21	0.01	0.02	0.02	0.25
Raddish red	0.21	0.01	0.02	0.01	0.25
Beet root	0.11	0.04	0.02	0.02	0.20
Onion white	0.11	0.01	0.01	0.02	0.15
Turnip	0.06	0.03	0.01	0.02	0.12
Sweet potato	0.06	0.01	0.02	0.02	0.12
Colocasia	0.06	0.01	0.01	0.02	0.11
Onion red	0.03	0.03	0.02	0.02	0.10
Yam	0.04	0.02	0.01	0.02	0.08
Potato	0.04	0.01	0.01	0.01	0.08
Garlic	0.02	0.02	0.01	0.02	0.07
Ginger	0.01	0.02	0.01	0.03	0.07

Table 7.16: Ranks based on relative contribution with respect to RDA

Fruit vegetables	*Zinc*	*Copper*	*Iron*	*Manganese*	*Selenium*	*Rank*
Brinjal green large	0.02	0.03	0.08	0.14	1.46	1.73
Ridge gourd	0.01	0.05	0.10	0.29	1.20	1.66
Tomato red	0.01	0.02	0.09	0.27	0.90	1.29
Tomato green	0.03	0.01	0.04	0.27	0.93	1.28
Red pumpkin	0.02	0.02	0.06	0.06	1.07	1.23
Brinjal purple	0.02	0.05	0.02	0.02	0.94	1.05
Ladies finger	0.01	0.01	0.08	0.12	0.75	0.98
Brinjal green small	0.02	0.04	0.04	0.08	0.66	0.83
Bitter gourd	0.02	0.01	0.05	0.31	0.36	0.76
Bottle gourd	0.01	0.01	0.02	0.04	0.57	0.65
Cauliflower	0.02	0.01	0.07	0.09	0.25	0.45
Coccinea	0.02	0.02	0.06	0.05	0.18	0.32
Capsicum	0.01	0.01	0.04	0.02	0.18	0.25
Mango ginger yellow	0.03	0.12	0.10	0.62	4.50	5.37
Turnip	0.01	0.07	0.09	0.67	3.10	3.94
Onion red	0.03	0.05	0.04	0.47	3.00	3.58
Ginger	0.04	0.12	0.02	0.85	2.10	3.14
Raddish red	0.01	0.12	0.09	0.58	2.30	3.11
Garlic	0.02	0.06	0.04	0.29	2.10	2.51
Carrot	0.03	0.10	0.05	0.49	1.50	2.16
Sweet potato	0.04	0.25	0.01	0.42	1.30	2.02
Onion white	0.01	0.06	0.03	0.38	1.30	1.78
Potato	0.01	0.05	0.01	0.40	1.30	1.77
Beetroot	0.01	0.02	0.07	0.29	1.30	1.69
Raddish white	0.01	0.09	0.02	0.04	1.40	1.55
Mango ginger white	0.07	0.06	0.01	0.47	0.60	1.21
Colocasia	0.03	0.10	0.01	0.20	0.50	0.83
Yam	0.03	0.12	0.01	0.25	0.20	0.61

Table 7.17: Bottom ranking fruits and vegetables based on MQI scores

0.1–0.2	*0.2–0.3*	*0.3–0.4*	*0.4–0.5*	*0.5–0.6*	*0.6–0.7*
Ziziphus big	Water chestnut	Tamarind white	Cauliflower	Tamarind red	Kokum
Water melon	Bottle gourd	Cabbage	Rose apple	Capsicum	Ambat chuka
Musk melon	Coccinea	Pear	Bel fruit	Papaya	Carrisa
Banana big	Tamarind	Custard apple	Tomato red	Brinjal purple	Coriander
Mint	Onion stalks	Patardi	Curry leaves	Onion white	
Apple		Gogu	Potato	Ladies finger	
Chikku		Cashew fruit	Lettuce	Bitter gourd	
Ziziphus small		Beet greens	Fenugreek	Safflower	
Banana small		Brinjal light green	Carrot greens	Sweet potato	
Ramphal		Keni	Ridge gourd	Pineapple	
		Ziziphus yellow	Tomato green		
		Knol-khol greens	Spinach		
			Red pumpkin		
			Pomegranate		
			Brinjal green		

Table 7.18: Top ranking fruits and vegetables based on MQI scores

0.7-0.8	*0.8-0.9*	*0.9-1*	*1 to 2*	*2 to 3*	*3 and above*
Mango ginger	Lemon	Colocasia black	Raddish white	Drumstick	Guava
Shepu		Mango alphanso	Garlic	Amaranth red	Raiamla
Onion red		Orange	Amaranth (viridis)	Big amla	
Haldi		Colocasia green	Strawberry		
Omum		Konphal	Wood apple		
Raddish red		Amaranth green	Raddish leaves		
Yam			Fetid cassia		
Carrot			Sweet lime		
Beet			Chakvat		
Ginger					
Colocasia green					

Table 7.19: Sample calculation in use of tables for computing contents of 8 micronutrients

Source	***% content***	***Asc acid***		***Beta carotene***		***Riboflavin***		***Thiamin***		***Zn***	***Cu***	***Fe***	***Mn***
	wt/100g prepared food	***raw mg %***	***cooked mg %***	***raw mcg %***	***cooked mcg %***	***raw mg %***	***cooked mg %***	***raw mg %***	***cooked mg %***	***mg %***	***mg %***	***mg %***	***mg %***
1. Spinach (ARI)	80	20.1	7.8	3368	60	0.12	0.08	0.03	0.03	0.17	0.05	0.8	0.51
Corn flour (NIN)	20	0		90		0.1		0.42		2.8	0.41	2.3	0.48
Spinach soup	100	0	6.24	18	48	0.02	0.064	0.084	0.024	0.696	0.122	1.1	0.504
Spinach soup			6.24		66		0.084		0.108	0.696	0.122	1.1	0.504
2. Spinach (ARI)	80	20.1	7.8	3368	60	0.12	0.08	0.03	0.03	0.17	0.05	0.8	0.51
Garlic (ARI)	10	1.75	0.63	45	8	0.019	0.013	0.024	0.015	0.69	0.26	0.53	4.7
Green chilli (NIN)	5	111		175		0.39		0.19		1.78	1.4	4.4	1.38
Lemon (ARI)	5	28		8		0.015		0.014		0.76	0.048	0.064	0.24
Spinach chutney	100	23.20		2708		0.118		0.037		0.332	0.138	0.916	0.959

Note: Raw and cooked values have been given only for vitamins and not for trace minerals. For calculation of spinach soup, the % contribution of each major ingredient is noted from recipe and cooked values of spinach are used. For spinach chutney all raw values are used. Readers may contact the authors to request for further assistance.

* ARI: Agharkar Research Institute, values estimated by us.

* NIN: National Institute of Nutrition, reposted values.

* Chutney: A spread of raw spinach made with ginger, green chillies, salt, lemon & cumin seeds.

REFERENCES

Henríquez-Sánchez P, Sánchez-Villegas A, Doreste-Alonso J, *et al*. 2009. Dietary assessment methods for micronutrient intake: a systematic review on vitamins. *Br J. Nutr.* 102(Suppl 1): S10–37.

Josep A, Dora R, and Antoni P 2005. The Diet Quality Index-International (DQI-I): is it a useful tool to evaluate the quality of the Mediterranean diet? *British Journal of Nutrition* 93: 369–376.

Kant AK, Schatzkin A, Graubard BI, and Schairer C 2000. A prospective study of diet quality and mortality in women. *Journal of the American Medical Association* 283: 2109–15.

Kennedy ET, Ohls J, Carlson S, and Fleming K 1995. The healthy eating index: design and applications. *Journal of the American Dietetics Association* 95: 1103–8.

Kune S, Kune GA and Watson LF 1987. Case-control study of dietary etiological factors: the Melbourne colorectal cancer study. *Nutrition and Cancer* 9(1): 21–42.

Lluýs SM, Lourdes R, and Joy N 2004. Food, youth and the Mediterranean diet in Spain. Development of KIDMED, Mediterranean Diet Quality Index in children and adolescents. *Public Health Nutrition* 7(7): 931–935.

McCullough ML, and Willett WC 2006. Evaluating adherence to recommended diets in adults: the Alternate Healthy Eating Index. *Public Health Nutr.* 9(1A): 152–7.

Tarwadi KV, and Agte VV 2005. Comparative performance of fruit and root vegetables with green leafy vegetables and fruits from Indian subcontinent for their antioxidant and micronutrient quality. *Journal of Science of Food and Agriculture* 85: 1469–1476.

Wahlqvist ML, Lo CS, and Myers KA 1989. Food variety is associated with less macrovascular disease in those with type II diabetes and their healthy controls. *Journal of the American College of Nutrition* 8(6): 515–23.

Annexures

Annexure-I

AVERAGE WEIGHTS OF STANDARD MEASURES FOR EACH COOKED FOOD ITEM

Food item	*Average serving measure*	*Weight (gms)*
Cereal preparations		
Chapati	One medium	45
Jawar roti	One medium	120
Bajara roti	One medium	60
Mix roti	One medium	75
Rice roti	One medium	80
Maize roti	One medium	80
Ragi roti	One medium	75
Green leafy vegetable preparations		
Cup (medium size, equivalent to 2 table spoons or small katori)		
Amaranthus red	Cup	60
Fenugreek and gram flour	Cup	100
Shepu	Cup	55
Onion stalks	Cup	100
Spinach	Cup	60
Raddish leaves	Cup	80
Gogu	Cup	110
Safflower	Cup	60
Corriander and gram flour	Cup	80
Fenugreek	Cup	60
Spinach cottage cheese	Cup	120
French beans carrot	Cup	120
Bittergourd	Cup	80
Bottle gourd	Cup	80
Capsicum	Cup	80
Cauliflower	Cup	80

Food item	***Average serving measure***	***Weight (gms)***
French beans	Cup	80
Knolkhol	Cup	80
Ladies finger	Cup	80
Tomato	Cup	80
Pumpkin	Cup	80
Ridge gourd	Cup	80
Snake gourd	Cup	80
Coccinea dry	Cup	80
Green tomato	Cup	80
Ash gourd	Cup	80
Yam	Cup	80
Brinjal	Cup	80
Field beans	Cup	80
Onion and gram flour	Cup	80
Potato	Cup	80
Potato onion	Cup	80
Radish	Cup	80
Drumstick curry	Cup	120
Sambhar	Cup	120
Carrot	Cup	80
Cucumber	Cup	80
Beet	Cup	80
Salads		
Carrot	Cup	80
Cucumber	Cup	80
Tomato	Cup	70
Cabbage	Cup	80
Cabbage + tomato + carrot	Cup	90
Carrot onion	Cup	85
Cucumber + curds	Cup	90
Onion greens	Cup	60
Knolkhol	Cup	105
Raddish	Cup	105
Beet	Cup	80
Fenugreek	Cup	80
Amaranthus red	Cup	80
Spinach	Cup	80
Lettuce	Cup	80
Fruits (edible portion)		
Apple	1	50
Banana ripe	1	80
Chikku	1	40
Guava	1	45
Mango ripe	1	100
Orange	1	35

Annexure-II

DESCRIPTION OF TRADITIONAL INDIAN FOOD ITEMS WITH THEIR MAIN INGREDIENTS

Item	*Description*	*Traditional name*
Cereal preparations		
Chapati	Unleavened whole wheat flour pan cake	Roti, Poli, Plain paratha
Jawar roti	Unleavened pan cake of whole jowar (sorghum) flour	Jowar bhakri
Bajara roti	Unleavened pan cake of whole bajara (pearl millet) flour	Bajra bhakri
Mix roti	Unleavened pan cake of whole wheat and bengalgram flour	Missi roti,
Rice roti	Unleavened rice flour pan cake	Rice bhakri
Corn roti	Unleavened pan cake of corn (maize) flour	Makai roti,
Ragi roti	Unleavened pan cake of ragi (finger millet) flour	Nachani bhakri
Green leafy vegetable preparations		
Red amaranth	Shallow fried red amaranthus coarsely cut, with tadka, onion	Lalmath subji
Fenugreek leaves and bengalgram flour	Shallow fried fenugreek leaves coarsely cut, with tadka, bengal gram flour, garlic	Methi subji
Shepu	Shallow fried fennel coarsely cut, with tadka, split green gram	Shepu subji
Onion stalks	Shallow fried onion stalks coarsely cut, with tadka	Kandapat subji
Spinach	Shallow fried spinach leaves coarsely cut, with tadka, onion	Palak subji
Raddish leaves	Shallow fried raddish leaves coarsely cut, with tadka, Bengal gram flour	Muli subji
Ambadi (Gogu)	Cooked gogu leaves coarsely cut, with Bengal gram flour, tadka, garlic	Gongura,
Safflower leaves	Shallow fried safflower leaves coarsely cut, with tadka, Bengal gram flour	Karadai subji
Corriander	Shallow fried coriander leaves coarsely cut, with tadka, onion	Dhania besan subji
Spinach leaves, cottage cheese	Cooked spinach leaves with cottage cheese cubes, tadka, garlic, ginger	Palak paneer curry
Spinach leaves	Cooked spinach leaves with tomato, onion, tadka, ginger	Palak tomato subji

Annexure-III

MICRONUTRIENTS IN HEALTH AND DISEASES

Micronutrients in Non Communicable Diseases

Supplementation of multivitamin and mineral supplement could reduce blood pressure and serum CRP in 128 Chinese women with increased cardiovascular disease risk.	Wang *et al.,* 2009
Favourable effect of vitamin E and selected carotenoids on gastric cancer and a detrimental effect of sodium even at intermediate levels of intake.	Pelucchi *et al.,* 2009
The risk of oral cavity cancer was determined in relation to serological levels of iron; vitamins A, B2, C, E; zinc; thiamin; and glutathione (GSH). Mild iron deficiency and low GSH levels, which are associated with increased oxidative stress, increase the risk of oral cavity cancer.	Richie *et al.,* 2008
The combination of diabetes and cataract coupled with gender bias and influence of socioeconomic factors seem to be associated with worsening of micronutrient status (selenium, zinc, iron, thiamine & vitamin A), oxidative stress, and lens opacity.	Agte and Tarwadi, 2008
Long-term multiple micronutrient supplementations can improve left ventricular volumes (LV) and LVEF and quality-of-life (QoL) scores in elderly patients with heart failure due to LV systolic dysfunction.	Witte *et al.,* 2005
Vitamins C and E, and lutein/zeaxanthin were ideal for ocular nutritional supplement	Bartlett and Eperjesi, 2004
The serum conc. of ascorbic acid was significantly (p<0.05) more reduced in pressure sore patients (mean+/-S.D.) 4.2+/-3.4 (ug/ml) than in control patients 7.4+/-5.4 (ug/ml) which still was lower than in a reference group (10.9+/-1.9) (ug/ml).	Selvaag *et al.,* 2002
Serum concentrations of several nutrients (beta-carotene, magnesium, selenium and zinc) were significantly lower in ulcerative colitis patients compared with controls. Serum vitamin B12 concentration was significantly lower in Crohn's disease patients.	Geerling *et al.,* 2000
More a micronutrient was correlated to total vegetable and fruit intake, the stronger was its protective effect against oral cancer.	Negri *et al.,* 2000
Supplementation with vitamin E, beta-carotene and selenium significantly decreased mortality rate from stomach cancer, primarily due to the decrease in deaths resulting from adenocarcinomas of the gastric cardia; it lowered the total mortality rate and showed signs of other beneficial effects.	Yang, 2000
Oral pre-cancerous lesions can certainly be reduced by beta-carotene, vitamin A, and other retinoids, and possibly by vitamin E. It also seems that retinoids can reduce pre-cancerous cervix, skin and lung lesions, that vitamin C and the NSAID sulindac can reduce colonic polyps, and that sunscreens can reduce solar keratoses.	Young and Lee, 1999

Micronutrients in Health – Adults

Prominent determinants of zinc status were intakes of beta-carotene and zinc along with environmental conditions and family size.	Agte *et al.,* 2005
Percentage of absorption of ascorbic acid showed weak positive associations with intakes of riboflavin (r=0.71) and ascorbic acid (r=0.5). There was a negative non-significant trend in values of beta-carotene absorption with increased intake of beta-carotene (r=-0.51, p>0.1) and iron (r=-0.67, P=0.1) but a positive significant trend with riboflavin intakes (r=0.84, P=0.018).	Agte *et al.,* 2005
Multiple regression analyses weighted for energy intake indicated a significant association of percent increase in Hb with intakes of iron, riboflavin, folic acid, beta-carotene, copper, phytate and fiber (p<0.01), percent change in plasma zinc with intakes of zinc, beta-carotene, vitamin C, riboflavin, copper, iron, and thiamin (p<0.01), percent change in vitamin C with intakes of vitamin C, vitamin E, niacin, riboflavin, thiamin, beta-carotene, zinc, phytate and fiber (p<0.05) and percent change in plasma beta-carotene with intakes of beta-carotene, thiamin, folic acid, zinc, phytate and tannins (p<0.05).	Agte *et al.,* 2006

Micronutrients in Health – Children and infants

A multiple micronutrient fortified diet for 6 months is more effective to improve the levels of hemoglobin, serum retinol, and RBP as well as to facilitate the mobilization of iron storage in preschool children than single micronutrient supplements.	Chen *et al.,* 2008
In 5- to 15-year-old children (n=281), nearly two-thirds were mildly riboflavin deficient. Riboflavin deficiency did not predict Hb and/or anaemia, but did predict iron deficiency among children free of malaria.	Rohner *et al.,* 2007
Supplementation with either zinc or iron decreased serum copper after 6 months in Bangladeshi infants.	Baqui *et al.,* 2005
Iron status was improved by daily multiple micronutrients (DMM) than daily placebo (P), weekly multiple micronutrient (WMM) or daily iron (DI) supplements in Vietnamese infants.	Hop le & Berger, 2005
The DMM was the most effective intervention tested, not only for improving anemia but also for improving iron, zinc, riboflavin, and tocopherol status in South African infants.	Smuts *et al.,* 2005
Although the DMM intervention was the most efficacious in Peruvian infants for preventing anemia, iron, and zinc deficiencies, 15%, 20%, and 50% of this group still remained anemic, zinc deficient, and iron deficient, respectively, at the end of the study. Further research thus should investigate whether higher doses of iron and zinc, together with infection control measures, are more efficacious.	López *et al.,* 2005

Table *(Contd...)*

Table *(Contd...)*

The DMM supplement was more efficacious than WMM or DI supplementation in improving infant status of other micronutrients, including zinc, tocopherol, and riboflavin, whereas DI exacerbated zinc deficiency. There were no significant differences in growth and morbidity among treatment groups, and growth faltering was not prevented in Indonesian infants.	Untoro *et al.*, 2005
In the pooled data, DMM was also the most effective treatment for controlling anemia and iron deficiency, besides improving zinc, retinol, tocopherol, and riboflavin status. Daily iron supplementation alone increased zinc deficiency.	Smut *et al.*, 2005
Iron and zinc administered together and with other micronutrients had a beneficial effect on infant motor development. Iron and zinc administered individually and in combination had a beneficial effect on orientation-engagement in Bangladeshi infants.	Black *et al.*, 2004
A 14 day course of zinc supplementation during acute shigellosis increased the lymphocyte proliferation and the Ipa-specific immunoglobulin G response.	Raqib *et al.*, 2004
Compared with control infants, infants whose mothers received FA alone or with iron or iron + zinc had a consistent pattern of 15–20% lower 3-month mortality in Nepal.	Christian *et al.*, 2003
Simultaneous supplementation of iron + zinc was associated with lower risk of severe diarrhea, 19% lower in all infants and 30% lower in less well-nourished infants with weight-for-age Z-score below-1. Iron + zinc supplementation was also associated with 40% lower risk of severe ALRI in less well-nourished Bangladeshi infants.	Baqui *et al.*, 2003
Zinc supplementation in 'small for gestational age infants' can result in a substantial reduction in infectious disease mortality.	Sazawal *et al.*, 2001
Infants fed Weanimix (a cereal-legume blend developed by the United Nations Children's Fund and the Ghanaian government) plus vitamins and minerals (WM) had better iron stores and vitamin A status than those fed nonfortified foods.	Lartey *et al.*, 1999

***In vitro* Models for Micronutrient Bioavailability**

Availability of non-heme iron for exclusively vegetarian meals has been associated with inositol diphosphate (IP), inositol penta phosphate (IP5), ascorbic acid, tannins, beta-carotene and hemicelluloses.	Chiplonkar & Agte, 2006
Bioavailable amount of zinc from vegetarian meals was influenced by IP3, IP5 and folic acid content and their interactive effect with zinc.	Chiplonkar & Agte, 2006
The *in vitro* zinc uptakes of erythrocytes in healthy subjects showed a strong negative correlation (p<0.01) with percent RBC hemolysis at 0.75,	Agte *et al.*, 2004

Table *(Contd...)*

Table *(Contd...)*

0.65 and 0.55% NaCl, a positive correlation with plasma zinc (r=0.33, p<0.05) and a strong negative correlation with plasma selenium and iron, hemoglobin and serum ceruloplasmin indicating antagonistic behavior of copper, iron and selenium with zinc uptake. Plasma ascorbic acid and status of riboflavin and thiamine were negatively correlated with *in vitro* zinc uptakes of erythrocytes in healthy subjects.	
At therapeutic zinc concentrations, folic acid and thiamine significantly enhanced the ABZn (p<0.010), while nicotinic acid inhibited zinc binding to albumin. Folic acid was found to enhance the ABZn also at lower zinc concentrations representing physiological levels of plasma zinc (138–150 micromoles) (p<0.05).	Agte & Nagmote, 2004
Under the zinc-deficient state, thiamine significantly enhanced the zinc uptakes by erythrocytes (p<0.05), whereas ascorbic acid and riboflavin inhibited zinc uptakes (p<0.05).	Agte *et al.*, 2004

Effects of Micronutrients

Dietary supplementation with vanadium, chromium, magnesium, zinc, selenium, copper and vitamins or cofactors (tocopherol [vitamin E], ascorbic acid [vitamin C], ubidecarenone [ubiquinone; coenzyme Q], nicotinamide, riboflavin, thioctic acid [lipoic acid] and flavonoids may be a complement to classical therapies for preventing and treating diabetic complications.	Bonnefont-Rousselot, 2004
Supplementation with vitamins A, C, E and Zn significantly reduced the micronucleus (MN) index by 13% (p=0.038). The results from this study illustrate the strong impact of a wide variety of micronutrients and their interactions on genome health, depending on the level of intake.	Fenech *et al.*, 2005
Adjunct therapy with zinc during acute shigellosis significantly improved seroconversion to shigellacidal antibody response and increased the proportions of circulating B lymphocytes and plasma cells.	Rahman *et al.*, 2005
The dietary intake of vitamin E, riboflavin, choline, magnesium, copper manganese and sulfur was significantly lower in patients of chronic pancreatitis than that of controls as well as the Recommended Dietary Allowance (RDA).	Bhardwaj *et al.*, 2004
Greater intake of dietary fiber, certain carotenoids, and vitamins may decrease the risk of esophageal adenocarcinoma, whereas greater intake of saturated fat may increase the risk of esophageal adenocarcinoma and distal stomach cancer.	Chen *et al.*, 2002

***In vivo* Models for Micronutrient Bioavailability**

Animal studies	Vitamin B2 had the strongest impact on liver Cu concentration in rats fed restricted diets.	Gralak *et al.*, 2004
	Single addition of Zn but not of methionine or riboflavin produced a growth response, but the combination of either Zn and Met or Zn and riboflavin resulted in growth responses that were greater than the response elicited by Zn alone.	Baker *et al.*, 1999
	There was significant improvement in the growth parameters like percent conception, mean weight gain in pregnancy, mean weight of pups at the age of 21 d, and percentage hemoglobin due to riboflavin supplementation ($p<0.05$). Percent zinc absorption, for the low-riboflavin diet, the supplemented diet, and the synthetic control diet were 16.4+/-5.7, 33.7+/-8.9, and 44.6+/-4.0, respectively, indicating the beneficial effect of riboflavin supplementation on iron and zinc utilization.	Agte *et al.*, 1998

References

Agte V, Jahagirdar M, and Chiplonkar S 2005. Apparent absorption of eight micronutrients and phytic acid from vegetarian meals in ileostomized human volunteers. *Nutrition* 21(6): 678–85.

Agte V, Jahagirdar M, and Chiplonkar S 2006. GLV supplements increased plasma beta-carotene, vitamin C, zinc and hemoglobin in young healthy adults. *Eur. J. Nutr.* 45(1): 29–36.

Agte VV, Chiplonkar SA, and Tarwadi KV 2005. Factors influencing zinc status of apparently healthy Indians. *J. Am. Coll. Nutr.* 24(5): 334–41.

Agte VV, Nagmote RV, and Chiplonkar SA 2004. Role of vitamin-zinc interactions on *in vitro* zinc uptake by human erythrocytes. *Biol. Trace Elem. Res.* 99(1–3): 99–112.

Agte VV, Nagmote RV, and Tarwadi KV 2004. Comparative *in vitro* uptake of zinc by erythrocytes of normal *vs* Type 2 diabetic individuals and the associated factors. *Diabetes Nutr. Metab.* 17(6): 343–9.

Agte VV, and Nagmote RV 2004. Study of factors affecting binding of zinc with albumin at physiological zinc concentrations. *Biofactors* 20(3): 139–45.

Agte VV, Paknikar KM, and Chiplonkar SA 1998. Effect of riboflavin supplementation on zinc and iron absorption and growth performance in mice. *Biol. Trace Elem. Res.* 65(2): 109–15.

Agte VV, and Tarwadi KV 2008. Combination of diabetes and cataract worsens the oxidative stress and micronutrient status in Indians. *Nutrition* 24(7–8): 617–24.

Baker DH, Edwards HM 3rd, Strunk CS, Emmert JL, Peter CM, Mavromichalis I, and Parr TM 1999. Single versus multiple deficiencies of methionine, zinc, riboflavin, vitamin B-6 and choline elicit surprising growth responses in young chicks. *J. Nutr.* 129(12): 2239–45.

for improving anemia, micronutrient status, and growth in South African infants. *J. Nutr*. 135(3): 653S–659S.

Smuts CM, Lombard CJ, Benadé AJ, Dhansay MA, Berger J, Hop le T, López de Romaña G, Untoro J, Karyadi E, Erhardt J, and Gross R 2005. International Research on Infant Supplementation (IRIS) Study Group. Efficacy of a foodlet-based multiple micronutrient supplement for preventing growth faltering, anemia, and micronutrient deficiency of infants: the four country IRIS trial pooled data analysis. *J. Nutr*. 135(3): 631S–638S.

Untoro J, Karyadi E, Wibowo L, Erhardt MW, and Gross R 2005. Multiple micronutrient supplements improve micronutrient status and anemia but not growth and morbidity of Indonesian infants: a randomized, double-blind, placebo-controlled trial. *J. Nutr.* 135(3): 639S–645S.

Wang C, Li Y, Zhu K, Dong YM, and Sun CH 2009. Effects of supplementation with multivitamin and mineral on blood pressure and C-reactive protein in obese Chinese women with increased cardiovascular disease risk. *Asia. Pac. J. Clin. Nutr*. 18(1): 121–30.

Witte KK, Nikitin NP, Parker AC, von Haehling S, Volk HD, Anker SD, Clark AL, and Cleland JG 2005. The effect of micronutrient supplementation on quality-of-life and left ventricular function in elderly patients with chronic heart failure. *Eur. Heart J*. 26(21): 2238–44.

Yang CS, 2000. Vitamin nutrition and gastroesophageal cancer. *J. Nutr*. 130(2S Suppl): 338S–339S.

Young KJ, and Lee PN 1999. Intervention studies on cancer. *Eur. J. Cancer Prev*. 8(2): 91–103.

Annexure-IV

BOTANICAL NAMES OF FRUITS AND VEGETABLES

Botanical Names of Green Leafy Vegetables

Name	*Botanical name*	*Name*	*Botanical name*
Chakvat	*Amaranthus paniculatus*	Tamarind	*Tamarindus indica*
Colocasia green	*Colocasia antiquorum*	Patardi	*Runcinata* D.C.
Fenugreek	*Trigonella foenum*	Curry leaves	*Murraya koenigii*
Shepu	*Pelargonium graveolens*	Red amaranth	*Amaranthus tricolor*
Mint	*Mentha spicata*	Drumstick	*Moringa oleifera*
Coriander	*Coriandrum sativum*	Colocasia black	*Colocasia antiquorum*
Spinach	*Spinacea oleracea*	Cabbage	*Brassica capitata*
Radish	*Raphanus sativus*	Onion stalks	*Allium cepa*
Gogu	*Hibiscus canabinus*	Carrot greens	*Daucus carota*
Ambat Chukka	*Rumex vesicarius*	Beet greens	*Beta vulgaris*
Cauliflower	*Brassica oleracea*	Omum leaves	*Trachyspermaum ammi*
Fetid cassia	*Cassia tora*	Garlic stalks	*Allium sativum*
Lettuce	*Lectuca sativa*	Knol khol leaves	*Brassica caulorapa*
Chavlai	*Amranthus viridis*	Keni	*Commenila enghalensis*
Safflower	*Carthamus tinctorius*		

Botanical Names of fruits

Guava	: *Psidium guajava*	Plum	: *Prunus persica*
Gooseberry	: *Emblica officinalis*	Pineapple	: *Ananas comoscus*
Cashew fruit	: *Anacardium occidentale*	Pomegranate	: *Punica granatum*
Bullock's heart	: *Annona reticulate*	Raisins	: *Vitis vinifera*
Apple	: *Malus sylvestris*	Rose apple	: *Syzygium jambos*
Pear	: *Persea Americana*	Sapota	: *Achras sapota*
Banana	: *Musa paradisiacal*	Custard apple	: *Annoma squamosa*
Bael fruit	: *Aegle marmelos*	Wood apple	: *Limonia acidissima*
Lemon	: *Citrus limon*	Zizyphus	: *Zizyphus jujube*
Sweet lime	: *Citrus sinensis*	Dates	: *Phoenix dactilifera*
Mango	: *Mangifera indica*	Kokum fruit	: *Garcinia indica*
Musk melon	: *Cucumis melo*	Tamarind	: *Tamarindus indica*
Water melon	: *Citrullus vulgaris*	Figs	: *Ficus carica*
Orange	: *Citrus aurantium*	Strawberry	: *Fragaria vesca*
Papaya	: *Carcia papaya*	Carissa	: *Carissa carandas*

Botanical Names of Fruit Vegetables and Root Vegetables

Fruit Vegetables		***Root Vegetables***	
Ladies fingers	: *Abelmoschus esculentus*	Onion	: *Allium cepa* (red and white)
		Potato	: *Solanum tuberosum*
Capsicum	: *Capsicum annum*	Beet root	: *Beta vulgaris*
Kovai	: *Ciccinia cordifolia*	Carrot	: *Dancus carota*
Tomato	: *Lycopersican esculentum*	Colocasia	: *Colocasia antiquorum*
		Mango ginger	: *Curcuma ameda* (white and orange)
Brinjal	: *Solanum melongena*		
Bitter gourd	: *Momordica charantia*	Garlic	: *Allium sativum*
Bottle gourd	: *Lagenaria vulgaris*	Ginger	: *Zinziber officinale*
Ridge gourd	: *Luffa accutangula*	Yam	: *Amorphophallus campanulatus*
Snake gourd	: *Trichosanthes anguina*	Sweet potato	: *Ipomoea batatas*
Pumpkin	: *Cucurbita maxima*	Tapioca	: *Manihot esculenta*
French beans	: *Phaseolus vulgaris*	Knol- khol	: *Brassica caulorapa*
Cluster beans	: *Cyamposis tetragonoloba*	Turnip	: *Brassica rapa*
		Radish	: *Raphanus sativus*

Annexure-V

ANTIOXIDANT POTENTIAL OF GREEN LEAFY VEGETABLES

Name	ITBARS mM Vit E/100 g		SOSA mM tannic acid/100 g		FICA mM EDTA/100 g		Polyphenols mg /100 g	
	Uncooked	Cooked	Uncooked	Cooked	Uncooked	Cooked	Uncooked	Cooked
Cabbage	0.67	0.38	21.93	11.75	26.95	19.56	40.1	34.3
Cauliflower	0.99	0.38	33.04	27.07	21.24	10.45	87	74.1
Onion stalks	0.61	0.37	38.5	29.4	32.8	23	65.26	54.29
Drumstick	0.71	0.36	30.55	28.75	65.4	29.4	163.9	154.1
Colocasia black	0.49	0.37	23.9	21.84	13.9	9.97	95.72	89.8
Colocasia green	0.22	0.36	55.9	5.87	55.91	50.64	80.5	74.5
Ambat chuka	0.6	0.38	28.63	17.64	23.71	23.88	105.63	95.8
Fetid cassia	0.76	0.34	23.1	12.13	21.1	14	121.82	111.25
Amaranthus green	0.62	0.38	13.9	5.5	13.9	7.09	127.6	109.62
Curry leaves	0.81	0.38	33.94	33.18	33.94	33.18	106.6	92.26
Fenugreek	1.01	0.38	41.16	24.45	35.4	13.42	55.8	50.24
Patardi	0.98	0.38	29.03	16.89	24.36	23.78	50.11	45.52
Tamrind	1.02	0.36	31.17	13.62	31.75	5.27	162.63	145.56
Amaranthus yellow	0.95	0.38	28.84	7.28	58.41	46.33	52.93	45.41
Shepu	0.76	0.38	16.89	4.66	47.14	30.55	124	119.26
Spinach	0.98	0.54	23.71	18.44	23.59	22.1	49.31	35.26
Amaranthus red	0.77	0.37	35.38	26.79	9.35	2.01	68.16	54.47
Safflower	0.75	0.39	33.13	9.33	35.3	26.75	123.2	112.38
Omum	0.86	0.38	55.91	29.12	29.2	18.6	240	239.11
Chakvat	0.6	0.38	34.07	21.21	36.21	36.64	45.45	36.54
Raddish	0.97	0.64	87.18	37.89	51.36	24.36	203.4	185.63
Gogu	0.48	0.38	34.07	8.49	52.94	46.95	108	95.45
Mint	0.61	0.38	10.64	2.98	1.82	0.86	36.67	25.59
Lettuce	0.73	0.21	47.07	30.22	43.78	21.67	62.3	54.47
Coriander	0.75	0.74	21.67	12.89	65.7	47.07	187.8	158.23
Keni	0.11	0.37	38.49	29.43	32.8	23.02	63.23	55.85
Knolkhol greens	0.45	0.2	23.9	8.5	28.45	10.1	112.4	99.65
Beet greens	0.26	0.09	30.2	9.3	30.7	19.7	84.5	76.64
Carrot greens	0.44	0.23	30	12.8	24.5	8.5	45.7	40.22

Levels of Vitamins in Green Leafy Vegetables

Name	*Ascorbic acid mg/100 g*		*Beta-carotene mg/100 g*		*Riboflavin mg/100 g*		*Thiamine mg/100 g*	
	Uncooked	*Cooked*	*Uncooked*	*Cooked*	*Uncooked*	*Cooked*	*Uncooked*	*Cooked*
Cabbage	6.5	2.1	488	240	0.1	0.1	0.02	0.01
Cauliflower	6.8	2.3	3112	60	0.13	0.1	0.05	0.02
Onion stalks	12.8	5.4	914	140	0.13	0.08	0.06	0.05
Drumstick	140	60.1	4944	200	0.03	0.03	0.02	0.02
Colocasia black	42.5	12	7072	240	0.1	0.08	0.03	0.03
Colocasia green	14	7.4	5678	240	0.14	0.1	0.05	0.03
Ambat chuka	8	4.3	2120	160	0.1	0.1	0.05	0.02
Fetid cassia	50.3	20.1		160	0.1	0.07	0.08	0.03
Amaranthus green	56	24.3	4144	200	0.11	0.1	0.04	0.03
Curry leaves	2.5	0.58	5208	160	0.1	0.07	0.08	0.03
Fenugreek	25.5	6.4	2008	160	0.09	0.05	0.07	0.03
Patardi	10.3	2.1	818	80	0.14	0.1	0.05	0.05
Tamrind	1.2	0.77		0	0.13	0.1	0.08	0.04
Amaranthus yellow	28	4.5	712	80	0.12	0.07	0.04	0.04
Shepu	16	3.3	4864	160	0.1	0.08	0.02	0.02
Spinach	20.1	7.8	3368	60	0.12	0.08	0.03	0.03
Amaranthus red	74	45.8	4764	160	0.09	0.05	0.07	0.03
Safflower	19.3	5.5	3304	80	0.11	0.07	0.05	0.03
Omum	21	10	2102	160	0.08	0.08	0.05	0.04
Chakvat	17.8	6.6	3104	160	0.12	0.1	0.08	0.04
Raddish	69.5	20.6	4648	160	0.11	0.11	0.03	0.03
Gogu	14.8	3.7	1338	160	0.11	0.1	0.04	0.04
Mint	1.4	0.52	899	160	0.09	0.07	0.03	0.02
Lettuce	4.8	1.3	944	80	0.1	0.1	0.03	0.02
Coriander	89.1	14.7	5064	80	0.05	0.04	0.04	0.03
Keni	12.8	5.4	322	40	0.1	0.08	0.06	0.05
Knol-khol greens	22.6	9.2	912	40	0.13	0.05	0.03	0.02
Beet greens	16.5	3.4	1026	160	0.11	0.08	0.04	0.02
Carrot greens	20.2	5.5	758	80	0.15	0.09	0.06	0.04

Levels of Trace Elements in Green Leafy Vegetables

Name	*Zinc mg/100 g*	*Copper mg/100 g*	*Iron mg/100 g*	*Manganese mg/100 g*	*Selenium mg/100 g*
Cabbage	0.01	0.01	0.78	0.04	0.21
Cauliflower	0.12	0.02	2.12	0.08	0.76
Onion stalks	0.03	0.02	1.06	0.04	0.42
Drumstick	0.1	0.03	8.34	0.04	0.51
Colocasia black	0.2	0.09	7.92	0.06	0.48
Colocasia green	0.05	0.05	8.1	0.05	0.5
Ambat chuka	0.16	0.04	5.84	0.04	0.76
Fetid cassia	0.08	0.02	12.9	0.04	0.51
Amaranthus green	0.13	0.07	2.1	0.04	0.5
Curry leaves	0.1	0.03	5.3	0.06	0.24
Fenugreek	0.09	0.03	1.5	0.08	0.32
Patardi	0.2	0.03	2.6	0.06	0.18
Tamrind	0.05	0.045	2.1	0.06	0.32
Amaranthus viridis	0.15	0.04	23.4	0.05	0.08
Shepu	0.1	0.04	10.9	0.04	0.4
Spinach	0.17	0.05	0.8	0.05	0.51
Amaranthus red	0.1	0.04	21.2	0.08	0.47
Safflower	0.09	0.04	4.7	0.08	0.76
Omum	0.08	0.03	6.6	0.08	0.34
Chakvat	0.07	0.03	28.7	0.05	0.88
Raddish	0.08	0.1	12.3	0.08	0.08
Gogu	0.08	0.04	2.12	0.05	0.01
Mint	0.08	0.01	0.55	0.02	0.03
Lettuce	0.07	0.03	3	0.04	0.76
Coriander	0.07	0.02	1.6	0.06	0.92
Keni	0.03	0.02	1.06	0.04	0.42
Knol-khol greens	0.06	0.01	1.15	0.04	0.25
Beet greens	0.09	0.09	1.77	0.02	0.19
Carrot greens	0.1	0.08	2.13	0.06	0.22

The significant correlations were found between

- ITBARS and SOSA (uncooked and cooked states) with selenium ($p<0.01$)
- SOSA uncooked state with SOSA cooked states with each other and with copper ($p<0.01$)
- FICA uncooked state and FICA cooked state with each other ($p<0.001$)
- Contents of zinc with contents of copper ($p<0.05$)
- Contents of polyphenols with SOSA, copper and selenium ($p<0.05$)

Antioxidant Potential of Fresh Fruits

Name	*ITBARS mM Vit E/100 g*	*SOSAmM tannic acid/ 100 g*	*FICAmM EDTA/100 g*	*Polyphenols mg/100 g*
Guava	0.97	34.35	47.8	97.8
Mango	0.28	19.13	31.1	39.8
Gooseberry small	0.8	47.8	30.5	1356
Gooseberry big	0.6	18.3	61.7	1324
Tamarind red	0.53	58.33	52.8	143.5
Tamarind white	0.29	35.37	38.7	81.9
Ziziphus big	0.22	35.74	35.05	195.8
Ziziphus small	0.61	16.24	33.8	49.6
Ziziphus yellow	0.16	35.75	39.3	37.8
Lemon	0.54	43.3	41.3	32.6
Sweet lime	0.23	45.9	28.9	40.6
Pineapple	0.28	28.74	46.9	101.5
Custard apple	0.67	34	45.7	53.6
Apple	0.61	25.5	56.7	142.1
Orange	0.3	16.32	33.2	77.5
Pomegranate	0.61	13.1	29.9	200
Rose apple	0.13	44.05	48.8	221.1
Banana big	0.59	14.65	9.3	50
Banana small	0.23	2.7	9.9	63.8
Kokum fruit	0.81	42.93	39.7	259.6
Carrisa	0.56	19.66	18.7	177.6
Papaya	0.3	30.32	40.7	86.3
Bullock's heart	0.49	27.9	33.7	39.15
Cashew fruit	0.67	54.16	49.1	49.31
Water chestnut	0.74	60.9	53.8	188.1
Bael fruit	0.19	77.19	62.4	104.4
Water melon	0.17	12.66	16.5	141.4
Musk melon	0.13	14.9	20.4	124.7
Sapota	0.24	11.67	15.1	23.9
Strawberry	0.36	22.68	18.6	54.4
Wood apple	0.34	28.54	20.7	167.5
Avocado pear	0.64	40.41	11.6	24.65

Levels of Vitamins in Fruits

Name	*Ascorbic acid mg/100 g*	*Beta-carotene mg/100 g*	*Riboflavin mg/100 g*	*Thiamine mg/100 g*
Guava	148	64	0.02	0.01
Mango	12	1200	0.10	0.02
Gooseberry small	325	16	0.02	0.02
Gooseberry big	345	16	0.02	0.03
Tamarind red	12	24	0.01	0.01
Tamarind white	8	24	0.01	0.01
Ziziphus big	1	24	0.01	0.01
Ziziphus small	3	16	0.02	0.01
Ziziphus yellow	8	24	0.02	0.01
Lemon	28	8	0.01	0.01
Sweet lime	41	40	0.02	0.01
Pineapple	16	32	0.16	0.04
Custard apple	10	24	0.03	0.02
Apple	5	8	0.01	0.02
Orange	33	24	0.04	0.03
Pomergranate	16	16	0.02	0.01
Rose apple	12	64	0.03	0.03
Banana big	4	16	0.01	0.02
Banana small	4	24	0.01	0.02
Kokum fruit	20	40	0.03	0.02
Carrisa	23	24	0.02	0.03
Papaya	16	48	0.01	0.01
Bullock's heart	3	64	0.02	0.02
Cashew fruit	10	56	0.02	0.03
Water chestnut	6	24	0.01	0.01
Bael fruit	12	8	0.02	0.03
Water melon	3	8	0.01	0.01
Musk melon	2	8	0.01	0.01
Sapota	4	54	0.01	0.01
Strawberry	41	56	0.02	0.03
Wood apple	44	64	0.03	0.02
Avocado pear	10	36	0.01	0.01

Levels of Trace Elements in Fresh Fruits

Name	*Zinc mg/100 g*	*Copper mg/100 g*	*Iron mg/100 g*	*Manganese mg/100 g*	*Selenium mg/100 g*
Guava	0.05	0.02	0.12	0.05	0.1
Mango	0.08	0.02	0.56	0.06	0.2
Gooseberry small	0.11	0.03	0.44	0.12	0.09
Gooseberry big	0.11	0.04	0.64	0.09	0.22
Tamarind red	0.04	0.04	0.40	0.16	0.08
Tamarind white	0.12	0.02	0.272	0.2	0.04
Ziziphus big	0.08	0.03	0.20	0.16	0.04
Ziziphus small	0.06	0.02	0.12	0.18	0.01
Ziziphus yellow	0.06	0.05	0.20	0.10	0.13
Lemon	0.07	0.01	0.04	0.08	0.03
Sweet lime	0.06	0.06	0.13	0.06	0.01
Pineapple	0.76	0.05	0.06	0.24	0.04
Custard apple	0.04	0.02	0.08	0.1	0.03
Apple	0.08	0.05	0.15	0.19	0.12
Orange	0.06	0.01	0.16	0.08	0.13
Pomegranate	0.02	0.05	0.20	0.03	0.06
Rose apple	0.10	0.06	0.32	0.16	0.08
Banana big	0.04	0.01	0.13	0.09	0.09
Banana small	0.05	0.02	0.08	0.2	0.13
Kokum fruit	0.07	0.01	0.26	0.24	0.07
Carrisa	0.05	0.01	0.11	0.09	0.02
Papaya	0.05	0.02	0.06	0.06	0.01
Bullock's heart	0.08	0.05	0.18	0.14	0.03
Cashew fruit	0.36	0.04	0.22	0.92	0.14
Water chestnut	0.31	0.05	0.34	0.64	0.05
Bael fruit	0.15	0.06	0.36	0.14	0.04
Water melon	0.06	0.02	0.04	0.12	0.02
Musk melon	0.06	0.04	0.03	0.04	0.04
Sapota	0.04	0.01	0.02	0.08	0.02
Strawberry	0.06	0.02	0.05	0.2	0.02
Wood apple	0.27	0.04	0.07	0.28	0.17
Avocado pear	0.09	0.02	1.48	0.44	0.04

Antioxidant Potential of Dry Fruits

Name	*ITBARS mM Vit E/100 g*	*SOSA mM tannic acid/ 100 g*	*FICA mM EDTA/100 g*	*Polyphenols mg/100 g*
Figs	0.48	60.84	48.97	249.4
Apricots	0.14	59.74	47.74	125.45
Dates	0.23	68.66	40.68	267.5
Plums	0.36	28.47	24.23	125.4
Raisins yellow	0.51	15.12	54.31	1364
Raisins dark	0.56	38.92	42.68	1278

Levels of Vitamins in Dry Fruits

Name	*Ascorbic acid mg/100 g*	*Beta-carotene mmg/100 g*	*Riboflavin mg/100 g*	*Thiamine mg/100 g*
Figs	2	24	0.11	0.12
Apricots	4	72	0.11	0.09
Dates	2	72	0.09	0.12
Plums	6	108	0.11	0.16
Raisins yellow	3	64	0.1	0.14
Raisins dark	5	64	0.11	0.13

Levels of Trace Elements in Dry Fruits

Name	*Zinc mg/100 g*	*Copper mg/100 g*	*Iron mg/100 g*	*Manganese mg/100 g*	*Selenium mg/100 g*
Figs	0.40	0.07	0.25	0.32	0.16
Apricots	0.31	0.06	0.34	0.10	0.17
Dates	0.52	0.06	0.37	0.12	0.15
Plums	0.16	0.04	0.18	0.08	0.12
Raisins yellow	0.50	0.03	0.82	0.50	0.08
Raisins dark	0.46	0.03	0.70	0.75	0.07

Comparisons for all the fruits revealed that

- The 3 antioxidant indices were strongly associated with each other ($p<0.001$).
- ITBARS were positively associated with selenium ($p<0.01$) while both SOSA and FICA had strong correlation with zinc ($p<0.001$).
- Copper was associated with zinc and manganese ($p<0.001$).
- Zinc was correlated with copper and manganese ($p<0.001$).
- Manganese was associated with zinc and copper ($p<0.001$) as well as with iron ($p<0.05$).
- Contents of polyphenols were associated with SOSA as well as selenium ($p<0.05$) and copper ($p<0.1$).

Antioxidant Potential of Fruit Vegetables

Name	*ITBARS mM Vit E/100 g*		*SOSA mM tannic acid/100 g*		*FICA mM EDTA/100 g*		*Polyphenols mg/100 g*	
	Uncooked	*Cooked*	*Uncooked*	*Cooked*	*Uncooked*	*Cooked*	*Uncooked*	*Cooked*
Brinjal	0.51	0.13	58.64	20.51	49.10	19.68	253.10	236.69
Snake gourd	0.48	0.16	50.55	19.68	46.05	11.64	145.70	123.25
Cluster beans	0.20	0.10	22.35	12.80	20.10	10.91	238.50	224.14
Tomato red	0.44	0.08	60.60	35.71	55.10	18.94	76.90	66.34
Tomato green	0.23	0.10	25.60	12.42	29.40	16.32	100.80	89.56
Ladies finger	0.67	0.21	37.70	11.88	43.30	20.15	128.30	101.14
Pumpkin	0.40	0.19	31.50	22.70	33.60	12.97	50.70	40.25
Bottle gourd	0.29	0.20	20.16	5.22	26.60	12.48	107.30	89.84
Bitter gourd	0.84	0.66	57.16	38.68	58.80	10.73	163.90	140.7
Ridge gourd	0.38	0.25	28.80	14.77	20.88	9.45	181.30	160.23
Coccinea	0.71	0.13	59.10	30.68	58.20	12.44	148.60	125.58
Capsicum	0.74	0.10	36.03	12.97	58.16	16.97	127.60	101.02

Levels of Vitamins in Fruit Vegetables

Name	*Ascorbic acid mg/100 g*		*Beta-carotene mg/100 g*		*Riboflavin mg/100 g*		*Thiamine mg/100 g*	
	Uncooked	*Cooked*	*Uncooked*	*Cooked*	*Uncooked*	*Cooked*	*Uncooked*	*Cooked*
Brinjal	3	1.12	58	12	0.04	0.03	0.02	0.01
Snake gourd	4.5	2.1	23	8	0.03	0.02	0.01	0.01
Cluster beans	7.5	4.3	50	18	0.04	0.02	0.02	0.01
Tomato red	18	7.58	33	12	0.02	0.02	0.03	0.02
Tomato green	13.5	9.21	49	12	0.01	0.01	0.02	0.01
Ladies finger	7.5	4.12	30	8	0.03	0.02	0.04	0.02
Pumpkin	5.3	2.56	25	9	0.02	0.01	0.05	0.04
Bottle gourd	3.5	1.85	20	4	0.02	0.01	0.02	0.01
Bitter gourd	59.5	11.48	51	14	0.03	0.02	0.02	0.01
Ridge gourd	9.3	4.47	11	4	0.02	0.01	0.04	0.02
Coccinea	7.8	4.15	70	24	0.02	0.01	0.02	0.01
Capsicum	83.5	13	183	80	0.02	0.01	0.02	0.02

Levels of Trace Metals in Fruit Vegetables

Name	*Zinc mg/100 g*	*Copper mg/100 g*	*Ironq mg/100 g*	*Manganese mg/100 g*	*Selenium mg/100 g*
Brinjal	0.22	0.11	2.74	1.62	0.12
Snake gourd	0.20	0.05	2.51	1.48	0.09
Cluster beans	0.25	0.03	2.07	0.52	0.03
Tomato red	0.34	0.05	1.59	0.34	0.11
Tomato green	0.29	0.08	1.14	0.43	0.07
Ladies finger	0.36	0.03	1.48	1.69	0.04
Pumpkin	0.41	0.03	1	1.50	0.09
Bottle gourd	0.32	0.04	1.57	0.27	0.02
Bitter gourd	0.22	0.03	2.23	0.66	0.08
Ridge gourd	0.34	0.07	2.1	0.77	0.15
Coccinea	0.1	0.03	0.52	0.20	0.06
Capsicum	0.11	0.02	1	0.10	0.02

Antioxidant Potential of Root Vegetables

Name	*ITBARS mM Vit E/100 g*		*SOSA mM tannic acid/100 g*		*FICA mM EDTA/100 g*		*Polyphenols mg/100 g*	
	Uncooked	*Cooked*	*Uncooked*	*Cooked*	*Uncooked*	*Cooked*	*Uncooked*	*Cooked*
Ginger	0.63	0.41	55.41	39.1	32.3	16.4	163	145.59
Garlic	0.44	0.27	48.66	33.15	52.4	29.78	184.9	170.49
Onion red	0.64	0.27	30.44	20.17	22.9	12.22	287.1	251.27
Onion white	0.57	0.26	19.68	9.2	20.6	11.19	118.2	95.94
Potato	0.38	0.17	11.4	7.1	14.11	5.69	170.4	144.58
Sweet potato	0.23	0.11	13.6	6.56	20.7	11.3	219.7	201.33
Radish white	0.78	0.58	51.21	25.84	40.19	14.11	166	145.6
Radish red	0.8	0.54	48.67	26.31	48.07	27.54	249.4	233.49
Colocasia	0.81	0.6	28.66	19.38	27.67	14.23	511.9	486.23
Yam	0.89	0.71	70.65	45.65	58.12	40.11	386.5	354.49
Tapioca	0.87	0.66	53.95	30.26	54.14	22.63	325.6	300.23
Beet-root	0.66	0.48	26.54	16.33	48.66	20.65	240.7	232.81
Mango ginger white	0.94	0.7	20.19	11.2	37.54	10.16	244.3	224.75
Mango ginger yellow	0.96	0.64	28.39	16.35	26.9	12.63	249.4	227.65
Carrot	0.78	0.33	36.2	11.16	28.35	9.85	60.18	45.88
Knol-khol	0.59	0.37	20.22	9.82	33.88	19.22	67.74	48.86
Turnip	0.54	0.29	31.67	13.65	23.41	9.55	107.71	89.59

Levels of Vitamins in Root Vegetables

Name	*Ascorbic acid mg/100 g*		*Beta-carotene mg/100 g*		*Riboflavin mg/100 g*		*Thiamine mg/100 g*	
	Uncooked	*Cooked*	*Uncooked*	*Cooked*	*Uncooked*	*Cooked*	*Uncooked*	*Cooked*
Ginger	1.33	0.45	40	8	0.02	0.01	0.03	0.02
Garlic	1.75	0.63	45	8	0.02	0.01	0.02	0.01
Onion red	3.88	1.25	76	24	0.03	0.02	0.02	0.01
Onion white	7.15	4.21	33	8	0.02	0.01	0.02	0.01
Potato	5.44	1.63	19	4	0.02	0.01	0.02	0.01
Sweet potato	6.32	2.58	28	8	0.03	0.02	0.02	0.01
Radish white	17.9	8.47	17	4	0.02	0.01	0.02	0.01
Radish red	19.3	8.45	14	4	0.03	0.02	0.02	0.01
Colocasia	6	2.56	33	8	0.02	0.01	0.02	0.01
Yam	4.9	1.47	49	12	0.01	0.01	0.02	0.01
Tapioca	5.84	2.36	78	24	0.02	0.01	0.02	0.02
Beet-root	9.37	4.58	94	26	0.03	0.01	0.03	0.01
Mango ginger white	20.85	9.54	68	24	0.03	0.01	0.02	0.01
Mango ginger yellow	23.8	10.05	63	24	0.02	0.01	0.02	0.01
Carrot	6.88	2.52	1237	648	0.02	0.02	0.03	0.01
Knol-khol	12	5.11	28	8	0.03	0.01	0.02	0.01
Turnip	39	15.69	9	0	0.03	0.02	0.02	0.01

Levels of Trace Elements in Root Vegetables

Name	*Zinc mg/100g*	*Copper mg/100g*	*Iron mg/100 g*	*Manganese mg/100g*	*Selenium mg/100g*
Ginger	0.64	0.55	0.23	2.3	0.13
Garlic	0.69	0.26	0.53	4.7	0.21
Onion red	1.1	0.13	0.31	2.6	0.06
Onion white	0.48	0.26	0.21	1.4	0.02
Potato	0.48	0.21	0.23	1.1	0.05
Sweet potato	0.23	0.1	0.2	2.2	0.13
Radish white	0.15	0.27	2.6	3.2	0.23
Radish red	0.15	0.13	0.8	2.1	0.13
Colocasia	0.16	0.15	2.6	3.7	0.31
Yam	0.42	0.21	1.33	2.7	0.15
Tapioca	0.45	0.26	2.9	3.4	0.45
Beet-root	0.4	0.1	1.13	2.6	0.3
Mango ginger white	0.15	0.05	2.0	1.6	0.13
Mango ginger yellow	0.26	0.13	1.13	1.6	0.21
Carrot	0.12	0.19	0.43	0.21	0.14
Knol-khol	0.21	0.09	0.65	0.22	0.11
Turnip	0.29	0.12	0.89	0.29	0.12

Comparisons by ANOVA of antioxidant indices and levels of micronutrients in cooked fruit vegetables (13) and root vegetables (15) with cooked GLV (30) and fresh fruits (30) revealed

- TBARS for all the 4 food groups to be significantly different ($F=6.35$, $p<0.05$)
- Significant differences for SOSA ($F=8.83$, $p<0.05$) and FICA (5.37, $p<0.05$)
- Non-significant difference in polyphenol contents ($F=1.55$)
- Significant difference in contents of beta-carotene ($F= 58.09$, $p<0.001$)
- A non-significant difference in contents of ascorbic acid ($F=1.07$)

Significant differences for contents of zinc ($F=16.52$, $p<0.01$) and selenium ($F=16.03$, $p<0.01$)

Comparison of Data with the Reported Values on 22 Common Foods

	ARI	*USDA*	*NIN*
Vitamin C (mg/100 g)			
Mean	8.86	12.51	13.87
SD	7.47	14.01	13.07
p value for t test	0.17	0.091	
Beta carotene (μg/100 g)			
Mean	591.1	1273.1	765.2
SD	1092.66	2366.4	1138.8
p value for t test	0.22	0.37	
Riboflavin (mg/100 g)			
Mean	0.033	0.045	0.065
SD	0.033	0.030	0.050
p value for t test	0.112	0.02	
Thiamine (mg/100 g)			
Mean	0.030	0.067	0.058
SD	0.027	0.050	0.040
p value for t test	0.005	0.011	
Zinc (mg/100 g)			
Mean	0.27	0.37	0.34
SD	0.23	0.73	0.47
p value for t test	0.31	0.28	
Copper (mg/100 g)			
Mean	0.083	0.085	0.18
SD	0.089	0.081	0.271
p value for t test	0.476	0.06	
Iron (mg/100 g)			
Mean	0.84	0.57	0.79
SD	1.09	0.64	0.52
p value for t test	0.165	0.416	
Manganese (mg/100 g)			
Mean	0.32	0.26	0.21
SD	0.42	0.31	0.19
p value for t test		0.33	0.23

Reference: USDA (FNB, 2001); NIN (2000)
* For majority of the comparisons, the differences were non-significant

Annexure-VI

METHODOLOGY FOR ASSESSMENT OF ANTIOXIDANT MICRONUTRIENT POTENTIAL

In vitro Methods for Assessment of Antioxidant Activity

Several of the commonly used methods for *in vitro* determination of antioxidant capacity are based either on biological oxidants (peroxyl radical, superoxide radical anion, hydrogen peroxide, hydroxyl radical, hypochlorous acid, singlet oxygen, nitric oxide radical, and peroxynitrite) or on non-biological assays (scavenging of 2,2'-azinobis-(3-ethylbenzo-thiazoline-6-sulphonate) radical cation (TEAC assay), scavenging of 2,2-diphenyl-1-picrylhydrazyl radical (DPPH assay), ferric reducing antioxidant power (FRAP assay), and the Folin-Ciocalteu reducing capacity (FC assay) (Schlesier *et al.,* 2002; Prior *et al.,* 2005; Huang *et al.,* 2005; Cao *et al.,* 1993; Ou *et al.,* 2001).

Depending upon the reactions involved, the assays for estimation of antioxidant activity can roughly be classified into two types: assays based on hydrogen atom transfer (HAT) reactions and assays based on electron transfer (ET) (Prior *et al.,* 2005). The majority of HAT-based assays apply a competitive reaction scheme, in which antioxidant and substrate compete for thermally generated peroxyl radicals through the decomposition of azo compounds. These assays include inhibition of induced low-density lipoprotein autoxidation, oxygen radical absorbance capacity (ORAC), total radical trapping antioxidant parameter (TRAP), and crocin bleaching assays. ET-based assays measure the capacity of an antioxidant in the reduction of an oxidant, which changes color when reduced. The degree of color change is correlated with the sample's antioxidant concentrations. ET-based assays include the total phenols assay (FC assay) by Folin-Ciocalteu reagent (FCR), Trolox equivalence antioxidant capacity (TEAC), ferric ion reducing antioxidant power (FRAP), "total antioxidant potential" assay using a Cu (II) complex as an oxidant, and DPPH. The Folin-Ciocalteu method is an ET based assay and gives reducing capacity, which has normally been expressed as phenolic contents (Huang *et al.,* 2005; Cao *et al.,* 1993; Ou *et al.,* 2001). The TEAC and the TRAP assays use the delay in oxidation and determine the lag phase as parameter for the antioxidant activity. They determine the delay of radical generation as well as the ability to scavenge the radical. In contrast, the assays DPPH, DMPD and FRAP analyze the ability to reduce the radical cation (DPPH, DMPD) or the ferric ion (FRAP) (Prior *et al.,* 2005).

One of the simplest methods of measurement of oxidative damage is lipid peroxidation. Lipid peroxidation refers to the oxidative degradation of lipids. It is the process whereby free radicals abstract electrons from the lipids in cell membranes, resulting in cell damage. This process proceeds by a free radical chain reaction mechanism. It most often affects polyunsaturated fatty acids, because they contain multiple double bonds. Certain diagnostic tests are also available for the quantification of the end products of lipid peroxidation, specifically malondialdehyde (MDA). The most commonly used test is called a TBARS Assay (thiobarbituric acid reactive substances assay).

On the whole, it can be supposed that results of various *in vitro* assays give an idea of the protective efficacy of secondary plant products. It is strongly recommended to use at least two methods due to the differences between the test- systems investigated (Prior *et al.,* 2005; Xianquan *et al.,* 2005; Rodriguez *et al.,* 2003; Reitveld *et al.,* 2003; Maiani *et al.,* 2008).

Procurement and processing

Among various fruits and vegetables available in the Indian markets, 15 root vegetables, 12 fruit vegetables, 30 fruits and 30 GLV were identified as the commonly consumed types. All the fruits and vegetables were procured from market fresh, cleaned with double distilled water and only the edible portions were collected. They were then homogenized in a blender to a uniform consistency.

Initially all the foods were analyzed for their antioxidant potential in the uncooked states. The effects of cooking and food processing are complex, as these processes can also vary the antioxidant potential in vegetables (Henry and Hepell, 2002). Hence for the estimations of the antioxidant activity and micronutrients in cooked states, the vegetables only (without any additions) were pressure cooked for 5 minutes at 15 lb. pressure and homogenized in a blender. The protocols followed are given below.

Inhibition of lipid peroxidation

MDA, formed from the breakdown of PUFA, reacts with thiobarbituric acid to give a red species absorbing at 528 nm. Inhibition of TBARS

chelating activity is high for compounds like EDTA and DTPA. Therefore EDTA was used as standard for this assay. Values were expressed as millimoles of EDTA equivalents per 100 g-food material.

Total phenolic contents

Reagents

(a) *Sodium bi-carbonate ($NaHCO_3$)*: 20% w/v in distilled water.

(b) *Folin-Ciocalteau reagent (FC reagent)*: 1mL of the reagent mixed with equal volume of water.

(c) *Standard gallic acid (0.1 mg/mL)*: Stock solution of gallic acid (1mg/mL in methanol) diluted suitably to obtain a working solution of 0.1 mg/mL.

(d) *Sample extracts*: 1g of food homogenate was extracted with 5 mL of water for 1 hour in an incubator-shaker maintained at 37°C.

The estimation was carried out as per the method described by Singleton *et al.*, (1965) and modified by Saucier *et al.*, (1999). For each analysis, sample extract as well as a series of standard solutions of Gallic acid were taken. Folin-Ciocalteau reagent was added to each tube and the solutions thoroughly mixed. After 30 seconds, $NaHCO_3$ solution was added. The tubes were left in dark at room temperature for 2 hours. The absorbance of the developed blue color was read at 700 nm. Values were expressed as milligrams per 100 g of Gallic acid.

Methods for assessment of micronutrients

Micronutrients were estimated spectrofluometrically/spectrophotometrically as per the methods described by Raghuramulu *et al.,* (2000).

Beta-carotene

The absorption of the reaction mixture at 460 nm is taken as the measure of beta-carotene in the sample.

Reagents

Alcoholic potassium hydroxide (KOH): 1 N KOH in 90% ethanol is prepared fresh and used for saponification.

Food sample was extracted with alcoholic KOH for 30 minutes. The extract was incubated in water-bath at 60°C for 20 minutes, removed and allowed to cool at room temperature. The unsaponifiable matter was then extracted 3 times with petroleum ether. The petroleum ether extract was washed with water to remove the alkali, passed through anhydrous sodium sulfate and evaporated to dryness under vacuum at 40µC. The dry residue was immediately dissolved in suitable amount of cyclohexane. The absorbance of cyclohexane solution, measured at 460 nm on a spectrophotometer gave the value of β-carotene content of the sample. The values were expressed as µg /100 g.

Ascorbic acid (vitamin C)

The blue color produced by the reduction of 2, 6 dichlorophenol indophenol dye by the ascorbic acid is estimated colorimetrically.

Reagents

(a) *Acetate buffer (pH 4.0)*: 33 g of anhydrous sodium acetate, 700 mL of water and 1000 mL glacial acetic acid are mixed.
(b) *Dye solution*: 2, 6 dichlorophenol indophenol (2,6 DCPIP) is dissolved in distilled water and made up to 200 mL.
(c) *Metaphosphoric acid (HPO_3)*: 6% w/v in distilled water.
(d) *Standard ascorbic acid*: 100 mg of pure ascorbic acid dissolved in 100 mL of 6% HPO_3.

Food sample was extracted with 6% HPO_3 for 30 minutes. The extract was drawn and acetate buffer was added to it. A sample blank and reagent blank (control) as well as standards were also simultaneously. The 2, 6 DCPIP dye solution was added in the control and sample tubes. The reduction of pink color of 2, 6-dichlorophenol by ascorbic acid was spectrophotometrically estimated at 520 nm. A standard curve was constructed and based on the average slope value the concentration of vitamin C was calculated. The values were expressed as mg/100g.

Riboflavin

The native fluorescence of riboflavin in neutral pH is used for the estimation of riboflavin.

Reagents

(a) *Potassium permanganate ($KMNO_4$)*: 4% w/v
(b) Caprylic alcohol

(c) *Hydrogen peroxide water mixture*: 1:1 v/v

(d) *Sodium hydroxide(NaOH)*: 0.1 M

(e) *Standard riboflavin solution*: 25 mg riboflavin dissolved in 200 mL water with 1.2 mL glacial acetic acid. The volume is made up to 1 L to get a stock solution of 25 µg/mL. The solution is suitably diluted to get a working solution of 1 µg/mL.

(f) *Sample extract*: Food sample was extracted with distilled water for 30 minutes.

To an aliquot of the sample extract, 1 drop of caprylic alcohol is added followed by $KMNO_4$ solution. The mixture was stirred and within 2 minutes, H_2O_2: H_2O mixture was added to discharge the permanganate color and pH adjusted to 7 with NaOH. The solution was filtered and fluorescence measured on a spectrofluorometer with excitation at 440 nm and emission at 640 nm. A series of riboflavin standards were also simultaneously run. The riboflavin content was calculated making due allowances for dilution and expressed as mg/100 g.

Thiamine

Estimation of thiamine is based on the oxidation of thiamine to thiochrome, which fluoresces in UV light. Under standard conditions and in the absence of other fluorescing substances, the fluorescence is proportional to the thiochrome present and hence to the content of thiamine.

Reagents

(a) *Basic lead acetate solution ($PbSO_4$)*: 180 g of $PbSO_4$ weighed and dissolved in 700 mL distilled water and the solution boiled. While boiling, 180 g lead oxide (litharge) is added and boiling continued for 30 minutes. The solution is made up to 1L after cooling.

(b) *Sodium hydroxide (NaOH)*: 40% w/v in distilled water with continuous shaking.

(c) *Potassium ferricyanide (K_3FeCN_6)*: 10% w/v in distilled water. Preserve in dark bottle in cold.

(d) Isobutyl alcohol

(e) *Sample extract*: Food sample was extracted with distilled water for 30 minutes.

(f) *Standard thiamine solution*: 25 mg of thiamine dissolved in 250 mL of 0.01 N HCl. 1 mL of this stock solution is diluted to 100 mL to get a working solution of 1 µg/mL.

To an aliquot of the sample extract, basic lead acetate solution was added and centrifuged. An aliquot of the same in another tube was treated with 30% H_2SO_4 and transferred to three, 100 mL separating funnels [1 serving as blank (B), 2 as experimental (E) and 3 as recovery (R)]. To all the three tubes, 40% NaOH was added. Solution of K_3FeCN_6 was added to E and R tubes and shaken well. To the R tube, 1mL of thiamine standard solution was added, mixed and allowed to stand for 2 minutes. Isobutyl alcohol was then added and mixed. The aqueous layer was rejected and the fluorescence of alcoholic layer was measured on a spectrofluorometer with excitation at 360 nm and emission at 485 nm. Thiamine content was calculated by the difference between the recovery (R) and experimental (E) and expressed as mg/100 g.

Levels of trace elements

Estimation is based on digestion of sample using a three acid mixture and reading the levels using atomic absorption spectrometry.

Reagents

(a) Nitric acid, Perchloric acid, Sulphuric acid in 3:2:1 proportion.

(b) *Standard solutions of trace elements*: Stock of 1000 ppm suitably diluted to get a series of working solutions in the range of 0.1 ppm-10 ppm.

(c) Metal free water (Millipore Q)

Dried food sample was accurately weighed and digested on a heating mantle using the 3 acid mixture. After diluting the sample suitably, analysis of trace metals such as zinc, copper, iron, manganese and selenium were carried out on Atomic Absorption Spectrophotometer (UNICAM, U.K.). Certified reference rice flour samples from National Institute of Environmental Sciences (NIES) were used as standards to check the precision and accuracy of the method. The measured concentrations of zinc, copper, iron, selenium and manganese were considered appropriate when they agreed well with the certified values.

Statistical methods

Mean and standard deviation for all the data were calculated. Differences between the antioxidant indices and micronutrients for four classes were compared using Student's t test and ANOVA. Paired t test was used for comparing data on uncooked and cooked forms of GLV, fruit vegetables and root vegetables. Correlations were computed as Pearson's correlation coefficient (r) using Excel for Windows 2000 and were considered significant for $p<0.05$.

REFERENCES

Cao G, Alessio H, and Cutler R 1993. Oxygen-radical absorbance capacity assay for antioxidants. *Free Radic. Biol. Med.* 14(3): 303–11.

Henry C, and Heppell N 2002. Nutritional losses and gains during processing: future problems and issues. *Proc. Nutr. Soc.* 61(1): 145–8.

Huang D, Ou B, and Prior RL 2005. The chemistry behind antioxidant capacity assays. *J. Agric. Food Chem.* 23; 53(6): 1841–56.

Maiani G, Periago Castón MJ, and Catasta G 2008. Carotenoids: Actual knowledge on food sources, intakes, stability and bioavailability and their protective role in humans. *Mol. Nutr. Food Res.* 53: Suppl2 5151–83.

Ou B, Hampsch-Woodill M, and Prior R 2001. Development and validation of an improved oxygen radical absorbance capacity assay using fluorescein as the fluorescent probe. *J. Agric. Food Chem.* 49(10): 4619–26.

Prior RL, Wu X, and Schaich K 2005. Standardized methods for the determination of antioxidant capacity and phenolics in foods and dietary supplements. *J. Agric. Food Chem.* 18; 53(10): 4290–302.

Raghuramulu N, Madhavan N and Kalyansundaram S 2000. *Ed*, A manual of laboratory techniques, National Institute of Nutrition, Hyderabad, India.

Rietveld A, and Wiseman S 2003. Antioxidant effects of tea: evidence from human clinical trials. *J. Nutr.* 133(10): 3285S–3292S.

Rodriguez-Amaya D, 2003. Food carotenoids: analysis, composition and alterations during storage and processing of foods. *Forum Nutr.* 56: 35–7.

Saucier C, and Waterhouse A 1999. Synergistic activity of catechin and other antioxidants. *J. Agri. Food Chem.* 47: 4491–94.

Schlesier K, Harwat M, Böhm V, and Bitsch R 2002. Assessment of antioxidant activity by using different *in vitro* methods. *Free Radic. Res.* 36(2): 177–87.

Singleton V, and Rossi J 1965. Colorimetry of total phenols with phosphomolybdic phosphotungstic acid reagents. *Am. J. Enol. Vitic.* 16: 144–158.

Williamson G, Susan M, Su W, *et al.* 1997. Induction of glutathione S transferase activity in hepG2 cells by extracts of fruits and vegetables. *Food Chem.*, 2: 157–160.

Xianquan S, Shi J, Kakuda Y, and Yueming J 2005. Stability of lycopene during food processing and storage. *J. Med. Food* 8(4): 413–22.

Yamaguchi F, Ariga T, Yoshimura Y, and Nakazawa H 2000. Antioxidative and antiglycation activity of garcinol from *Garcinia indica* fruit rind. *J. Agri. Food Chem.* 48: 180–185.

Annexure-VII

REVIEW OF LITERATURE ON DEVELOPMENT OF QUALITY INDEX

Nutritional rating systems are techniques of ranking individual foods, food products or food categories to evaluate the nutritional quality of food. The systems may use point as a basis to rank or rate foods for general nutritional value or they may rate specific food attributes such as cholesterol content. Graphics or other symbols can be used to communicate the scores to the target population. Nutritional rating systems differ from nutritional labeling in the sense that they attempt to simplify food choices, and do not list specific amounts of nutrients or ingredients. Dietary guidelines and the nutritional rating systems both attempt to simplify the communication of nutritional information, however, they do not rank individual food products.

There is a report of Overall Nutritional Quality Index (ONQI) as an algorithm designed by a team of experts by Dr. Katz (http://www.nuval.com/Science/origins) to generate a single, summative score for the "overall nutritional quality" of a food based on its micronutrient and macronutrient composition and several other of its nutritional properties (*e.g.*, energy density). The ONQI is claimed further to be designed to stratify foods into a rank order of relative nutrition potential both universally (*i.e.* for all food categories) and within specific food categories (*e.g.*, breads, cereals, frozen desserts, etc.). It avoids the characterization of any food as "good" or "bad" in absolute terms. ONQI is an algorithm which converts complex nutritional information into a single, easy-to-use score and which defines the nutritional quality of foods based on the influence they have on overall dietary goals. Factors included in developing ONQI were fiber; folate; vitamins A, C, D, E, B12, B6; potassium; calcium; zinc; omega 3 fatty acids; bioflavanoids; carotenoids; magnesium; iron; saturated fat; trans fat; sodium; sugar; cholesterol; fat quality; protein quality; energy density and glycemic load. But, the ONQI is based on a patent-pending concept not freely available and not useful for other countries and there is need to develop a quality index for Indian foods. Secondly, there has not been a quality index for antioxidant quality.

There have been reports about overall diet quality to be associated with chronic disease risk and health outcomes (Kant *et al.,* 2000; Jacques and Tucker, 2001). McCullough *et al.* (2002) found that high scores on

Subject Index

B

C

P

Q

R

S

T